Psychosocial Palliative Care

Psychosocial Palliative Care

William S. Breitbart, MD

Interim Chairman
Chief, Psychiatry Service, Department of Psychiatry
and Behavioral Sciences
Attending Psychiatrist, The Palliative Medicine Service
Department of Medicine, Memorial Sloan-Kettering Cancer Center
Professor of Clinical Psychiatry, Department of Psychiatry
Weill Medical College of Cornell University
New York, New York

Yesne Alici, MD

Assistant Attending Psychiatrist
Memorial Sloan-Kettering Cancer Center
Assistant Professor of Psychiatry
Weill Medical College of Cornell University
New York, New York

OXFORD
UNIVERSITY PRESS

OXFORD
UNIVERSITY PRESS

Oxford University Press is a department of the University of
Oxford. It furthers the University's objective of excellence in research,
scholarship, and education by publishing worldwide.

Oxford New York
Auckland Cape Town Dar es Salaam Hong Kong Karachi
Kuala Lumpur Madrid Melbourne Mexico City Nairobi
New Delhi Shanghai Taipei Toronto

With offices in
Argentina Austria Brazil Chile Czech Republic France Greece
Guatemala Hungary Italy Japan Poland Portugal Singapore
South Korea Switzerland Thailand Turkey Ukraine Vietnam

Published in the United States of America by
Oxford University Press
198 Madison Avenue, New York, NY 10016

Library of Congress Cataloging-in-Publication Data
Breitbart, William, 1951– author.
Psychosocial palliative care / William S. Breitbart, Yesne Alici ; with the International
Psycho-Oncology Society.
p. ; cm.
Includes bibliographical references and index.
ISBN 978–0–19–991740–2 (print : alk. paper) —
ISBN 978–0–19–936632–3 (e-book) — ISBN 978–0–19–936633–0 (e-book)
I. Alici, Yesne, author. II. International Psycho-Oncology Society,
sponsoring body. III. Title.
[DNLM: 1. Palliative Care—psychology. 2. Palliative Care—methods.
3. Terminally Ill—psychology. WB 310]
R726.8
616.02'9—dc23
2013042001

9 8 7 6 5 4 3 2
Printed in the United States of America
on acid-free paper

Contents

Preface

The International Psycho-Oncology Society (IPOS) established the IPOS Press in 2006, during my tenure as a member of the IPOS executive board. An IPOS Press task force, led by Drs. Maggie Watson, Luigi Grassi, and myself nurtured the IPOS Press throughout the subsequent years, as each of us on the IPOS Press task force had the honor to serve IPOS for 2-year terms as IPOS president. (My tenure as president was from 2008 to 2010.) In 2006 and 2008, IPOS Press collaborated with the American Psychosocial Oncology Society to produce the first of two Pocketbook Quick Reference Guides for psycho-oncology clinicians, with pharmaceutical industry support. The two Pocketbooks included a: (1) *Quick Reference Guide for Oncology Clinicians: the Psychiatric and Psychosocial Dimensions of Cancer Symptom Management*; and (2) *Quick Reference for Pediatric Oncology Clinicians: The Psychiatric and Psychological Dimensions of Pediatric Cancer Symptom Management*. (See www.ipos-society.org for more information on ordering these pocket reference books.) *Psychosocial Palliative Care* represents the latest in a series of IPOS texts to be published through IPOS Press, and we are quite excited about the variety of clinical and research-oriented books we anticipate will be available to the oncology and psycho-oncology communities over the next years.

Psychosocial Palliative Care had a long journey to publication which began in 2007. My clinical, research, and writing career had steadily moved from general psycho-oncology, toward a focus on the interface of psycho-oncology and palliative care. This transition was brought into being by several events and opportunities. In 1995 I was selected to be in the first US national cohort of Soros Faculty Scholars of the Open Society Institute, Project on Death in America, which supported by research activities in psychosocial palliative care for the next 3 years. This experience solidified my identity as a psychiatric palliative care clinician as well as a psycho-oncologist. Subsequently I co-edited, with Dr. Harvey Chochinov the first and second editions of the *Handbook of Psychiatry in Palliative Medicine*, by Oxford University Press. In 2002, I took on the role of editor-in-chief of Cambridge University Press's international palliative care journal, *Palliative & Supportive Care*. Now in its 11th year of continuous publication, *Palliative & Supportive Care* remains the only international palliative care journal that focuses on the psychiatric, psychosocial, existential, and spiritual domains of palliative care. The actual genesis of *Psychosocial Palliative Care* took place in 2004, when I was asked by my good friend, Dr. James Levenson to write the chapter on palliative care for the first major comprehensive textbook in *Psychosomatic Medicine*[1] that was to serve as the reference textbook for all subspecialty board certification questions on the examination for subspecialty certification in psychosomatic medicine in the United States. As you can imagine, I had a sense of profound responsibility to an entire subspecialty field of psychiatry, and I was compelled to write the ultimate, most comprehensive chapter on palliative care and its psychiatric and psychosocial dimensions ever written! Well, I went a bit overboard, and submitted a chapter that was 175 pages long and contained 800 references. It was a book, not a chapter. My dear editor and friend, Jim Levenson, was very kind to me. He wrote me a simple email; "Bill, great chapter. Very comprehensive. I will go over the chapter and edit it so that it is an appropriate length to be included in the textbook." The edited, shortened chapter was approximately one-fourth the length and scope of what I had submitted. Surprisingly, it reads quite well. However, I realized that I indeed had written a small textbook. At this time we were developing the concept of establishing an IPOS Press as a means for IPOS members to publish textbooks, but through a publishing mechanism that would bring much-needed revenue to IPOS in order to fulfill its mission. I submitted a slightly revised version of my original chapter as a small book for consideration by the IPOS task force for publication. I received much helpful feedback about a variety of elements of what I had originally produced: (1) a briefer, more succinct format, with less text and more tables in order to match the first IPOS Quick Reference Guides; (2) a more international perspective on palliative care and especially cultural issues and sensitivities; and so on. Over the next year I undertook the task of adapting what I had produced to match the IPOS Quick Reference Guide format. This adaptation was accomplished primarily by the dedicated and brilliant work of two medical students who spent elective time with me at Memorial Sloan-Kettering. Gloria Chansong Lee, MD, was the first to transform the massive text into the Quick Reference Guide format. Anna Lopatin Dickerman, MD, spent an entire summer refining the book and updating my original references. This task was completed in 2007, but unfortunately IPOS Press could not find financial support to publish this Pocket Handbook. Oxford University Press (OUP) came to the rescue. Abby Gross, our incredible OUP editor on the IPOS Press/Oxford University Press publication of *Dr. Holland's Textbook of Psycho-oncology*, 2nd ed, saw the potential for an IPOS Press–Oxford University Press collaboration in producing this *IPOS Pocket Handbook for Clinicians* dedicated to psychosocial aspects of palliative care. Andrea Seils has deftly taken over editorial and publisher responsibility for this project from Abby Gross, and we are so appreciative of her guidance and support. What remained, before actual publication, was the massive task of updating all the contents of the textbook since 2007. This was a challenging and important job made more difficult by the fact that there has been an explosion of important new epidemiological, correlative, and intervention studies in the literature in just the past several years alone. My colleague and coauthor, Dr. Yesne Alici, took on the task of this update, and even initiated an expansion into areas that had not been originally included in the earlier version of the text because of advances made in the field.

During a 30-year career in psycho-oncology, I have learned that everything takes at least three times longer than you thought it would. We have exceeded that dictum. However, I learned an even greater lesson from my mother that gives me comfort when I think of the very long and difficult journey on which this project has taken me. My mother was a Holocaust survivor and lived a difficult early life. However, she persevered and survived long enough to experience a long life blessed with many joys to complement the tragedies through which she lived. During challenging and difficult times my mother often reminded me of our ethnic and family legacy, saying, "Things always come very hard for us my son, but in the end, when they appear, the taste is much sweeter!" Perhaps it is fitting that a text on the psychosocial aspects of palliative care can serve as an example that out of hardship and suffering, beauty and meaning can be derived, and savored, perhaps even for generations.

William Breitbart, MD

Reference

1. Breitbart W, Gibson C, Chochinov H. Palliative care. In: Levenson JL, ed. *The American Psychiatric Publishing Textbook of Psychosomatic Medicine*. Washington, DC: American Psychiatric Publishing; 2004:979–1007.

Introduction

One of the most challenging roles for clinicians working in the cancer setting is to help guide advanced and terminally ill cancer patients and their families through the physical, psychological, and spiritual aspects of the dying process. Patients with cancer and other life-threatening illnesses are at increased risk for the development of major psychiatric complications, and have an enormous burden of both physical and psychological symptoms.[1,2] In fact, surveys suggest that psychological symptoms such as depression, anxiety, and hopelessness are as frequent, if not more so, than pain and other physical symptoms.[3–5] Concepts of adequate palliative care must be expanded beyond the current focus on pain and physical symptom control to include the psychiatric, psychosocial, existential, and spiritual aspects of care. The psycho-oncologist, as a consultant to or member of a palliative care team, has a unique role and opportunity to fulfill this promise of competent and compassionate palliative care for those with life-threatening illness. Oncologists and palliative care physicians, as well as oncology and palliative care nurses, as the central members of the multidisciplinary palliative care team, must also develop the knowledge and skills necessary to work collaboratively and provide comprehensive palliative care, which includes the psychiatric, psychosocial, existential, and spiritual domains of palliative care.

This pocket handbook guides the psycho-oncologist and palliative care clinician through the most salient aspects of effective psychiatric and psychosocial care of patients with advanced illness. We review basic concepts and definitions of palliative care; a global perspective on death and palliative care; the assessment and management of major psychiatric complications of life-threatening illness, including psychopharmacological and psychotherapeutic approaches; and issues such as bereavement, spirituality, cultural sensitivity, communication, and psychosocial contributions to the control of common physical symptoms.

It is important to note that the *Diagnostic and Statistical Manual of Mental Disorders*, 5th ed. (DSM-V)[6] was released in May 2013 for use by mental health professionals in the United States. Because there is much controversy[7] around its implementation in clinical care and research, we have decided to continue using the *Diagnostic and Statistical Manual of Mental Disorders*, 4th ed, Text Revision (DSM-IV-TR)[8] in this handbook until the DSM-V becomes more widely accepted in the medical community.

When caring for patients with advanced cancer, AIDS, or other illnesses, the focus of treatment may often shift to symptom management and the enhancement of quality of life. Such patients are uniquely vulnerable to both physical and psychiatric complications. The high prevalence of distressing physical symptoms, such as pain, makes the assessment of psychiatric symptoms difficult. The role of the psycho-oncologist in the care of the terminally ill or dying patient is critical to both adequate symptom control and integration of the physical, psychological, and spiritual dimensions of human experience throughout the course of illness and especially near the end of life.

References

1. Breitbart W, Chochinov H, Passik S. Psychiatric symptoms in palliative medicine. In: Hanks G, Cherny N, Christakis N, eds. *Oxford Textbook of Palliative Medicine*, 4th ed. New York: Oxford University Press; 2010:933–956.
2. Chochinov HMC, Breitbart W, ed. *Handbook of Psychiatry in Palliative Medicine*, 2nd ed. New York: Oxford University Press; 2009.
3. Portenoy RK, Thaler HT, Kornblith AB, et al. The Memorial Symptom Assessment Scale: An instrument for the evaluation of symptom prevalence, characteristics, and distress. *Eur J Cancer* 1994;30A:1326–1336.
4. Vogl D, Rosenfeld B, Breitbart W, Thaler H, Passik S, McDonald M, et al. Symptom prevalence, characteristics and distress in AIDS outpatients. *J Pain Symptom Manage*. 1999;18:253–262.
5. Gao W, Bennett MI, Stark D, Murray S, Higginson IJ. Psychological distress in cancer from survivorship to end of life care: prevalence, associated factors and clinical implications. *Eur J Cancer* 2010;46(11):2036–2044.
6. American Psychiatric Association. *Diagnostic and Statistical Manual of Mental Disorders*, 5th ed. Arlington, VA: American Psychiatric Publishing; 2013:5–25.
7. Transforming diagnosis by Thomas Insel, MD. http://www.nimh.nih.gov/about/director/2013/transforming-diagnosis.shtml. Accessed July 14, 2013.
8. *Diagnostic and Statistical Manual of Mental Disorders*, 4th ed., text rev. Washington, DC: American Psychiatric Association; 2000.

Part I

Modern Palliative Care

Chapter 1

Principles of Palliative Care

Defining Palliative Care

The terms "palliative care" and "palliative medicine" are often used interchangeably. Palliative medicine refers to the medical discipline of palliative care, an approach to improve the quality of life of patients who are facing life-threatening illness and their families.[1,2,3] Modern palliative care has evolved from the hospice movement into a more expansive network of clinical care delivery systems with components of home care and hospital-based services.[4] The nature and focus of palliative care has similarly evolved over the century, expanding beyond the concept of comfort care for only the dying. This care may begin with the onset of a life-threatening illness and proceeds past death to include bereavement interventions for family and others (Figure 1.1). Introduction of palliative care shortly after diagnosis to patients with metastatic non-small cell lung cancer has been shown to result in better quality of life and lower rates of depression.[5] Palliative care must meet the needs of the "whole patient"—and his or her family—while addressing physical, psychological, social, spiritual, and existential aspects of suffering (Box 1.1).[4,5]

The Global Need for Palliative Care

It is estimated that 33 million dying people worldwide are in need of palliative care.[4] When one considers the additional burden affecting family members of the seriously ill, this estimate grows to 100 million people. Moreover, the population of aging and chronically ill individuals continues to grow. Despite the global emergence of modern hospice and palliative care over the past 50 years, barriers to adequate care persist. These include unequal access to care, insufficient funding, and lack of national policies.[6] Worldwide, but especially

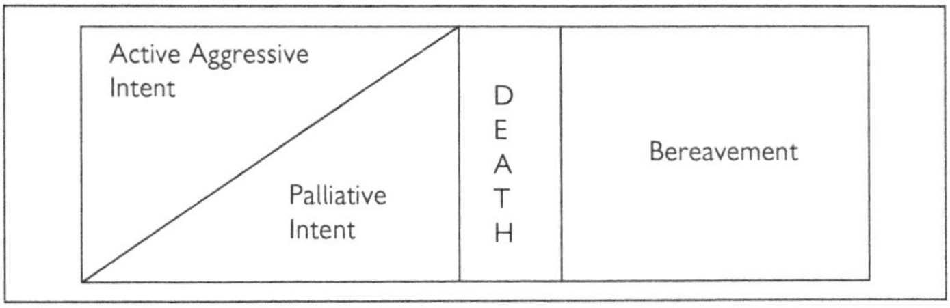

Figure 1.1 Current Model of Palliative Care

Box 1.1 World Health Organization Definition of Palliative Care[1,2]

Palliative care:

- Provides relief from pain and other distressing symptoms
- Affirms life and regards dying as a normal process
- Intends neither to postpone nor hasten death
- Integrates the psychological and spiritual aspects of patient care
- Offers a support system to help patients live as actively as possible until death
- Offers a support system to help the family cope during the patient's illness and in their own bereavement
- Uses a team approach to address the needs of patients and their families, including bereavement counseling, if indicated
- Will enhance the quality of life, and may also positively influence the course of illness
- Is applicable early in the course of illness, in conjunction with other therapies that are intended to prolong life, such as chemotherapy or radiation therapy
- Includes the investigations needed to better understand and manage distressing clinical complications

in developing countries, most cancers are incurable at the time of diagnosis. Curative treatments are often available or of minimal benefit, yet palliative care can provide pain relief and symptom management for the vast majority of such patients. In developing countries, where palliative care is often unavailable, this continues to be a challenge (Boxes 1.2 and 1.3).[4]

Today, more than 8,000 hospice and palliative care initiatives exist worldwide in more than 100 countries (www.hospiceinformation.info).[6] These include inpatient units, hospital-based services, community-based teams, day care centers, and other modes of delivery (Box 1.4).

Palliative Care Programs/Models of Care Delivery

Palliative care is not restricted to those who are dying or those enrolled in hospice programs, but rather, can be applied to the control of symptoms and

Box 1.2 Estimated Number of People in Need of Palliative Care (in millions)[4]

Annual deaths globally	56
Annual deaths in developing countries	44
Annual deaths in developed countries	12
Estimated numbers needing palliative care globally*	33

* It can be estimated that approximately 60% of the dying need palliative care

Box 1.3 2nd Global Summit of NHPCA* Declaration on Hospice and Palliative Care, March 2005[7]

- Governmental health policy should include palliative care (as recommended by WHO).
- Access to palliative care should be considered a human right.
- Resources should be available for hospice and palliative care programs and services.
- Necessary drugs should be made available (including affordable and available morphine for the poorest).
- Hospice and palliative care should be available to all citizens in the setting of choice—acute care hospitals, long-term care facilities, residential hospices, and patients' homes.

* National Hospice and Palliative Care Association.

provision of support to those living with chronic, life-threatening illnesses. Palliative care is a relatively inexpensive and efficient means of controlling pain and physical symptoms, and meeting the needs of those nearing the end of life.[6,13–15] Indeed, palliative care for individuals with AIDS and cancer has been instituted as national policy in countries that are neither wealthy nor industrialized. Uganda's inclusion of palliative care in its National Health Plan for 2000–2005, for example, demonstrates the effectiveness of an integrated government and community nongovernmental approach to palliative care.[4]

Fully developed, model, palliative care programs ideally include all of the components listed in Box 1.5. The model of care delivery is interdisciplinary.

Palliative Care Does Not Hasten Death

Physicians, patients, and family members often believe that the transition from curative to palliative care (e.g., discontinuing antitumor-focused treatments, initiating treatments for symptom control and comfort) results in shorter survival time. This concern often leads to a delay in initiating palliative care and perhaps the unnecessary continued use of less than beneficial antitumor treatments.[17,18] There is also a common concern that medications, such as opioids used for pain, may unintentionally hasten death in patients receiving palliative care in settings such as palliative care units, hospice units, or home hospice care.[19,20]

A 2007 study by the National Hospice and Palliative Care Organization[21] examined survival rates in approximately 5,000 cancer patients with advanced disease. Hospice patients receiving palliative treatment survived an average of 29 days longer than those who did not receive hospice care. This study[21] further supports that medications for symptom relief, such as high doses of morphine and other opioids, do not hasten death. Other recent studies have also demonstrated that the aggressive use of opioids and sedatives to provide "sedation" for the control of pain and other symptoms in terminally ill cancer patients is not associated with shorter survival (Box 1.6).[22–25]

Box 1.4 Estimated Statistics on Hospice and Palliative Care

Americas

- United States[7,8]
  - More than 5,300 hospices serving approximately 1,650,000 patients
  - Nearly one in five agencies with a dedicated inpatient unit/facility
  - More than 1,000 hospital-based pain and palliative care services
  - 64 academic medical school affiliated departments of palliative medicine
  - 85 pain and palliative medicine fellowship training programs offering more than 234 fellowship positions
  - Several major national palliative care organizations, and more than 10 national and international palliative care scientific journals published
- Canada: more than 600 palliative care services[12]
- Costa Rica: 26 palliative care clinics[7]
- Argentina: 30 palliative care and supportive care teams
- Uruguay: 17 palliative care services

Europe

- Central/Eastern Europe: 466 organizations[10]
- Western Europe[11]
  - Belgium: 152 organizations
  - Germany: 706 organizations
  - Italy: 91 organizations
  - Netherlands: 338 organizations, 72 palliative networks
  - Romania: 25 palliative care services
  - Spain: 144 organizations
  - United Kingdom: 1,158 organizations

Asia Pacific[9]

- Hong Kong: 15 organizations
- India: 49 organizations
- Japan: 102 organizations
- Korea: 28 organizations
- Taiwan: 28 organizations
- China: 20 organizations*
- Vietnam: 5 organizations
- Singapore: 10 organizations
- Philippines: 16 organizations
- New Zealand: 38 organizations
- Australia: 230 organizations

Africa and Middle East

- Sub-Saharan Africa: 16 organizations
- South Africa: 6 palliative care teams

* 2011 statistics report approximately 150 hospice/palliative care services in China[30].

Box 1.5 Ideal Components of a Palliative Care Program[12]

1. A home care (e.g., hospice) program
2. A hospital-based palliative care consultation service
3. A day care program or ambulatory care clinic
4. A palliative care inpatient unit or dedicated palliative care hospital beds
5. A bereavement program
6. Training and research programs
7. Internet-based services

In the 2010 study by Temel and colleagues,[5] patients assigned to early palliative care had a better quality of life than did those assigned to standard care. In addition, fewer patients in the palliative care group than in the standard care group had depressive symptoms (16% vs. 38%, $p = .01$). Despite the fact that fewer patients in the early palliative care group than in the standard care group received aggressive end-of-life care (33% vs. 54%, $p = .05$), median survival was longer among patients receiving early palliative care (11.6 months vs. 8.9 months, $p = .02$).

Psycho-oncologists helping palliative care teams, patients, and families make decisions around the transition from curative to palliative care can now present strong evidence that a decision to choose palliative care and utilize opioids or sedatives will not result in hastening the death process. Thus, greater acceptance as well as less fear of palliative care may result in earlier and more

Box 1.6 Palliative Care Does NOT Hasten Death[5,16–25]

- Palliative care does not hasten death. In a 2007 study, terminally ill patients receiving hospice care were observed to survive longer than non-hospice patients[21].
- A 2010 study by Temel and colleagues[5] showed that among patients with metastatic non-small cell lung cancer, early palliative care led to significant improvements in both quality of life and mood. As compared with patients receiving standard care, patients receiving early palliative care had less aggressive care at the end of life but longer survival.
- There have been additional studies to define[26] "early palliative care" and study[27–29] the impact of early palliative care on the quality of life, symptom burden, and survival. There is no doubt that early palliative care improves quality of life and reduces symptom burden at the end of life.
- Use of opioids/sedative medications for symptom relief does not hasten death.
- Hospice care enhances social support for patients and families, and may be an influence in survival effects of aggressive palliative care.

frequent utilization of palliative care interventions. This can not only result in better symptom control, but also facilitate discussion of existential issues that confront those facing the end of life.

References

1. World Health Organization. *National Cancer Control Programmes: Policies and Managerial Guidelines*, 2nd ed. Geneva: World Health Organization; 2002.
2. World Health Organization. *Cancer Control: Knowledge into Action. Palliative Care: WHO Guide for Effective Programmes*. Geneva: World Health Organization; 2007.
3. Sepulveda C, Marlin A, Yoshida T, Ullrich A. Palliative care: the World Health Organization's global perspective. *J Pain Symptom Manage*. 2002;24:91–96.
4. Stjernsward J, Clark D. Palliative medicine: a global perspective. In: Doyle D, Hanks G, Cherny N, Calman K, eds. *Oxford Textbook of Palliative Medicine*, 3rd ed. New York: Oxford University Press; 2004:1199–1224.
5. Temel JS, Greer JA, Muzikansky A, Gallagher ER, Admane S, Jackson VA, et al. Early palliative care for patients with metastatic non-small-cell lung cancer. *N Engl J Med*. 2010;363(8):733–742.
6. Help the Hospices. Hospice and palliative care worldwide: the need for palliative care. http://www.helpthehospices.org.uk/about-hospice-care/international/ Accessed July 10, 2013.
7. McDermott E. *Advocating hospice and palliative care: challenges, contexts and changes*. The 2nd Global Summit of National Hospice and Palliative Care Associations. Seoul, Korea, 2005.
8. National Hospice and Palliative Care Organization. Facts on hospice and palliative care. http://www.nhpco.org/files/public/Statistics_Research/2012_Facts_Figures.pdf Accessed July 14, 2012.
9. Goh CR. The Asia Pacific Hospice Palliative Care Network: a network for individuals and organizations. *J Pain Symptom Manage*. 2002;24:128–133.
10. Clark D, Wright M. *Transitions in End of Life Care: Hospice and Related Developments in Eastern Europe and Central Asia*. Buckingham, UK: Open University Press; 2003.
11. Have H, Clark D. *The Ethics of Palliative Care: European Perspectives*. Buckingham, UK: Open University Press; 2002.
12. Fainsinger RL. Canada: palliative care and cancer pain. *J Pain Symptom Manage*. 2002;24(2):173–176.
13. Bruera E, Neumann CM, Gagnon B, Brenneis C, Quan H, Hanson J. The impact of a regional palliative care program on the cost of palliative care delivery. *J Palliat Med*. 2000;3(2):181–186.
14. Raftery JP, Addington-Hall JM, MacDonald LD, Anderson HR, Bland JM, Chamberlain J, et al. A randomized controlled trial of the cost-effectiveness of a district co-ordinating service for terminally ill cancer patients. *Palliat Med*. 1996;10(2):151–161.
15. Fassbender K, Fainsinger R, Brenneis C, Brown P, Braun T, Jacobs P. Utilization and costs of the introduction of system-wide palliative care in Alberta, 1993-2000. *Palliat Med*. 2005;19(7):513–520.
16. Breitbart W, Chochinov H, Alici Y. End-of-life care. In: Grassi L, Riba M, eds. *Clinical Psycho-oncology: An International Perspective*. Oxford, UK: Wiley; 2012:249–270.

17. Miyashita M, Sanjo M, Morita T, Hirai K, Kizawa Y, Shima Y, et al. Barriers to providing palliative care and priorities of future actions to advance palliative care in Japan: a nationwide expert opinion survey. *J Palliat Med.* 2007;10(2):390–399.

18. Christakis NA, Escarce JJ. Survival of Medicare patients after enrollment in hospice programs. *N Engl J Med.* 1996;18:335(3):172–178.

19. Krakauer EL, Penson RT, Truog RD, King LA, Chabner BA, Lynch TJ. Sedation for intractable distress of a dying patient: acute palliative care and the principle of double effect. *Oncologist* 2000;5(1):53–62.

20. Cavanaugh TA. The ethics of death-hastening or death-causing palliative analgesic administration to the terminally ill. *J Pain Symptom Manage.* 1996;12:248–254.

21. Connor SR, Pyenson B, Fitch K, Spence C, Iwasaki K. Comparing hospice and nonhospice patient survival among patients who die within a three-year window. *J Pain Symptom Manage.* 2007;33:238–246.

22. Morita T, Tusunoda J, Ihoue S, Chihara S. Effects of high dose opioids and sedatives on survival in terminally ill cancer patients. *J Pain Symptom Manage* 2001;(21)4:282–289.

23. Vitetta L, Keaner D, Serli A. Sedation and analgesia-prescribing patterns in terminally ill patients at the end of life. *Am J Hospice Palliat Med.* 2005;22:465–473.

24. Bercovitch M, Adunsky A. Patterns of high-dose morphine use in a home-care hospice service: should we be afraid of it? *Cancer* 2004;101:1473–1477.

25. Sykes N, Thorns A. Sedative use in the last week of life and the implications of end-of-life decision making. *Arch Intern Med.* 2003;163:341–344.

26. Yoong J, Park ER, Greer JA, Jackson VA, Gallagher ER, Pirl WF, et al. Early palliative care in advanced lung cancer: a qualitative study. *JAMA Intern Med.* 2013;173(4):283–290. doi: 10.1001/jamainternmed.2013.1874.

27. Irwin KE, Greer JA, Khatib J, Temel JS, Pirl WF. Early palliative care and metastatic non-small cell lung cancer: potential mechanisms of prolonged survival. *Chron Respir Dis.* 2013;10(1):35–47. doi: 10.1177/1479972312471549.

28. Pirl WF, Greer JA, Traeger L, Jackson V, Lennes IT, Gallagher ER, et al. Depression and survival in metastatic non-small-cell lung cancer: effects of early palliative care. *J Clin Oncol.* 2012;30(12):1310–1315.

29. Greer JA, Pirl WF, Jackson VA, Muzikansky A, Lennes IT, Heist RS, et al. Effect of early palliative care on chemotherapy use and end-of-life care in patients with metastatic non-small-cell lung cancer. *J Clin Oncol.* 2012;30(4):394–400. doi: 10.1200/JCO.2011.35.7996. Epub December 27, 2011.

30. China Daily (2011) Families lament lack of palliative care centers. http://www.chinadaily.com.cn/cndy/2011-03/29/content_12240782.htm Accessed March 29, 2011.

Chapter 2

A Global Perspective on Death

To understand and treat psychiatric issues in the dying patient today, psycho-oncologists must have an appreciation of why, when, where, and how patients die in the third millennium.

Causes of Death

Whereas some common causes of death can be sudden (e.g., myocardial infarction, stroke, gunshot wound), others, such as cancer and human immunodeficiency virus (HIV) disease, have become chronic diseases. These chronic illnesses often have a prolonged dying process that may necessitate psychiatric intervention and treatment (Boxes 2.1 and 2.2).

Age of Death

The mean life expectancy in the United States as of 2010 was 78.2 years. Life expectancy is similar in other industrialized regions of the world, illustrating the importance of care for elderly and dying individuals. At the other end of the spectrum, life expectancy is greatly reduced to the third and fourth decade in sub-Saharan Africa. This is largely because of the impact of poverty and infectious diseases such as HIV/AIDS.[1] Clearly, there is a broad range of life expectancies throughout the world. For a comprehensive list, see the World Health Organization's World Health Statistics, 2012 at http://www.who.int/gho/publications/world_health_statistics/2012/en/index.html.

Box 2.1 Leading Causes of Death Worldwide, 2011[1]

1. Ischemic heart disease
2. Stroke and other cerebrovascular disease
3. Lower respiratory infections
4. Chronic obstructive pulmonary disease
5. Diarrheal diseases
6. HIV/AIDS
7. Trachea, bronchus, and lung cancers
8. Tuberculosis
9. Diabetes mellitus
10. Road traffic accidents

Box 2.2 Leading Causes of Death in the United States, 2011[2]

1. Diseases of the heart
2. Malignant neoplasms
3. Chronic lower respiratory diseases
4. Cerebrovascular diseases
5. Accidents (unintentional injuries)
6. Alzheimer's disease
7. Diabetes mellitus
8. Influenza and pneumonia
9. Nephritis, nephritic syndrome, and nephrosis
10. Intentional self-harm (suicide)
11. Septicemia
12. Chronic liver disease and cirrhosis
13. Essential hypertension and hypertensive renal disease
14. Parkinson's disease
15. Pneumonitis resulting from solids and liquids

Location of Death

These trends indicate that health care workers should be well educated about, and experienced with, end-of-life issues, including psychiatric issues (Box 2.3).

How Do Patients Die?

It appears that many patients do not die "good" deaths, but rather "bad" deaths, characterized by needless suffering and disregard for patients' or families' wishes and/or values (Box 2.4).

Box 2.3 Patient Preferences on Location of Death

- Studies have found that around 75% of respondents would prefer to die at home.
- Between 50% and 70% of people receiving care for advanced illness would prefer home care at the end of life.
- Despite the preference for home care and death at home, only 20% to 30% of individuals in the United States and Western Europe ultimately die at home.
- Death in hospital remains common in many countries[3].
- A retrospective cohort study[4] of Medicare beneficiaries aged 66 and older compared sites of death, place of care, and rates of health care transitions in 2000, 2005, and 2009. Although there was a lower proportion who died in an acute care hospital in 2009 (24.6%) and 2005 (26.9%) compared with 2000 (32.6%) both intensive care unit (ICU) use (29.2% in 2009, 26.3% in 2005, and 24.3% in 2000) and the rate of health care transitions increased in the last month of life. In the same retrospective cohort, 43.4% of cancer patients died at home in 2009 compared with 41.5% of patients in 2000.

Box 2.4 The Patient's Death[5]

- A technological imperative characterizes Western medical practice, including care of the dying.
- Substantial shortcomings exist in the care of seriously ill hospitalized patients.
  - poor communication between physicians and dying patients
  - implementation of overly aggressive treatment, often against patients' wishes
- There is a need for greater skills and education in end-of-life issues.
- There is a need for increased communication with and support of dying patients.

What Is a "Good" Death?

Clearly, each individual has his or her own definition of a good death. Culturally specific communities and rituals influence communal approaches to dying and suffering (Box 2.5).[9]

These four criteria and the aforementioned considerations for achieving a good death can serve as general guidelines for the psycho-oncologist in caring for the dying (Box 2.6).

Box 2.5 World Health Organization Guidelines for a "Good" Death[6–8]

- A "good" death is one that
  - is free from avoidable distress and suffering for patient, family, and caregivers
  - is in general accord with the patient's and family's wishes, and
  - is reasonably consistent with clinical, cultural, and ethical standards.

Box 2.6 Weisman's Four Criteria for an "Appropriate Death"[10]

1. Internal conflicts, such as fears about loss of control, should be reduced as much as possible.
2. The individual's personal sense of identity should be sustained.
3. Critical relationships should be enhanced or at least maintained, and conflicts resolved, if possible.
4. The person should be encouraged to set and attempt to reach meaningful goals, even though limited (e.g., attending a graduation, a wedding, or the birth of a child), as a way to provide a sense of continuity into the future.

References

1. World Health Organization. The top 10 causes of death. http://www.who.int/mediacentre/factsheets/fs310/en/index.html Accessed July 14, 2013.
2. Centers for Disease Control and Prevention. Deaths: preliminary data for 2011. *Natl Vital Stat Rept.* 2011;61(6). http://www.cdc.gov/nchs/data/nvsr/nvsr61/nvsr61_06.pdf Accessed July 14, 2013.
3. World Health Organization. Palliative care: the solid facts. http://www.euro.who.int/__data/assets/pdf_file/0003/98418/E82931.pdf Accessed July 14, 2013.
4. Teno JM, Cozalo PI, Bynum JP, et al. Change in end-of-life care for Medicare beneficiaries: site of death, place of care, and health care transitions in 2000, 2005, and 2009. *JAMA.* 2013;309(5):470–477.
5. SUPPORT Principal Investigators. The Study to Understand Prognoses and Preferences for Outcomes and Risks of Treatments (SUPPORT): a controlled trial to improve care. *JAMA.* 1995;274:1591–1598.
6. World Health Organization. *Cancer pain relief and palliative care: report of a WHO expert committee (technical bulletin 804).* Geneva: World Health Organization; 1990.
7. World Health Organization. *Cancer pain relief and palliative care: report of a WHO expert committee (technical bulletin 804)*, 2nd ed. Geneva: World Health Organization; 1996.
8. World Health Organization. *Symptom relief in terminal illness.* Geneva: World Health Organization; 1998.
9. Koffman J, Crawley L. Ethnic and cultural aspects of palliative care. Section 3.7. In: Hanks G, Cherny N, Christakis A, Fallon M, Kaasa S, Portenoy RK, eds. *Oxford Textbook of Palliative Medicine*, 4th ed. New York: Oxford University Press; 2010.
10. Weisman AD. *On Dying and Denying: A Psychiatric Study of Terminality.* New York: Behavioral Publications; 1972.

Chapter 3

Role of the Psycho-oncologist in Palliative Care

The psycho-oncologist's role in the care of the dying patient is essential and diverse. The psycho-oncologist can participate in pain and symptom management through the use of pharmacological and nonpharmacologic adjunctive therapies.[1–3] A primary role of psycho-oncologists is the diagnosis and treatment of comorbid psychiatric disorders that may complicate the course of a life-threatening illness. The role of the psycho-oncologist in the care of the dying extends beyond the management of psychiatric symptoms and syndromes into areas that include existential issues, family and caregiver support, bereavement, doctor-patient communication, education, and training (Box 3.1).[4,5]

Box 3.1 Role of the Psycho-oncologist in Palliative Care

- Diagnosis and treatment of comorbid psychiatric disorder (e.g., delirium, depression, anxiety disorders; see chapters 4–8)
- Helping the patient deal with the existential crisis posed by a terminal diagnosis
- Helping families cope with anticipatory grief and other strong emotions that surround the imminent death of a loved one (this may include, but is not limited to, the provision of psychotherapeutic interventions)
- Assisting with management of social, psychological, ethical, legal, and spiritual issues that complicate the care of dying patients
- Exploring treatment options (e.g., palliative care, alternative treatments, participation in experimental clinical trials, maximal comfort care)
- Serving as an advocate for the patient as questions arise about insurance, coverage of home health aides, and eligibility for home care services
- Enlisting pastoral involvement, when appropriate
- Assisting conflict resolution among patient, family, and staff by opening lines of communication
- Facilitating the process of end-of-life discussions and decision making, including:
  1. Encouraging discussion about end-of-life decisions regarding treatment, withholding resuscitation, and life support
  2. Encouraging appointment of a health care proxy
  3. Providing psychiatric evaluation of patient's capacity to make rational judgments and the proxy's ability to make an appropriate decision for the patient
  4. Providing psychiatric consultation for maximal comfort, if needed[6]

(continued)

Box 3.1 (Continued)

- Providing continued support to family and other loved ones during the bereavement period
- Educating medical staff about psychological issues involved in the care of dying patients, including:
  1. Physical and psychological symptom management
  2. Effective communication with dying patients
  3. Discussions about prognosis and do not resuscitate (DNR) orders

References

1. Cassem NH. The dying patient. In: Hackett TP, Cassem NH, eds. *Massachusetts General Hospital Handbook of General Hospital Psychiatry*, 2nd ed. Littleton, MA: PSG Publishing; 1987:332–352.
2. Cassell E. *The Nature of Suffering and the Goals of Medicine*. New York: Oxford University Press; 1991.
3. Breitbart W, Levenson JA, Passik SD. Terminally ill patients. In: Breitbart W, Holland JC, eds. *Psychiatric Aspects of Symptom Management in Cancer Patients*. Washington, DC: American Psychiatric Press; 1993:173–230.
4. Breitbart W, Holland JC, eds. *Psychiatric Aspects of Symptom Management in Cancer Patients*. Washington, DC: American Psychiatric Press; 1993.
5. Chochinov HM, Breitbart W, eds. *Handbook of Psychiatry in Palliative Medicine*, 12th ed. New York: Oxford University Press; 2012.
6. Subcommittee on Psychiatric Aspects of Life-Sustaining Technology. The role of the psychiatrist in end-of-life treatment decisions. In: *Caring for the Dying: Identification and Promotion of Physician Competency (Educational Resource Document)*. Philadelphia, PA: American Board of Internal Medicine; 1996:61–67.

Part II

Psychiatric Disorders in the Palliative Care Setting

Patients with advanced disease, such as advanced cancer, are particularly vulnerable to psychosocial concerns, psychiatric disorders, and complications.[1–5] Incidences of pain, depression, and delirium increase with higher levels of physical debilitation and advanced illness. Psychological symptoms such as worrying, nervousness, lack of energy, insomnia, and sadness are among the most prevalent and distressing in these populations.[6] Neuropsychiatric symptoms and syndromes such as mood disorders (depression), cognitive impairment disorders (delirium), anxiety, insomnia, and suicidal ideation coexist with many other physical and psychological symptoms and interact with each other, negatively affecting quality of life.

Psychological symptoms and psychiatric disorders must be understood in the context of the patient and family as the unit of concern. Prompt recognition and effective treatment of both psychiatric and physical symptoms is critically important to the well-being of the patient with advanced disease and to the well-being of his or her family. Physicians caring for terminally ill patients must develop their skills in assessment and management of psychiatric symptoms and disorders.

Strategies for Psychiatric/Psychological Symptom Control in the Terminally Ill

Psychiatric/psychological symptom control in patients with advanced disease can be understood and approached in a fashion similar to physical symptom control.[3]

Two Strategies for Psychiatric/Psychological Symptom Control in Dying Patients
1. A management approach focusing on symptoms as opposed to syndromes:
• Use of psychotropic agents to treat symptoms rather than specific syndromes (e.g., antidepressants for neuropathic pain, insomnia, appetite; atypical antipsychotics for insomnia, nausea, anxiety, appetite)
2. A syndrome-based approach:
• Use of psychotropic agents to treat a specific identifiable syndrome (e.g., antidepressants for depressive disorders, benzodiazepines for anxiety disorders)
• Challenging, partly because the origin of such symptoms may be caused by advanced medical illness, medical treatments, or a psychiatric syndrome

The psycho-oncologist must incorporate both approaches, depending on the specific clinical presentation.

Chapters 5, 6, 7, and 8 describe the prevalence, assessment and management of the most common psychiatric disorders encountered in the palliative cancer care setting: anxiety disorders, depression, suicide and suicidal ideation, and delirium.

References

1. Breitbart W, Marotta RF, Call P. AIDS and neuroleptic malignant syndrome. *Lancet*. 1988;21:488–1489.
2. Breitbart WS, Alici Y. Psycho-oncology. *Harv Rev Psychiatry*. 2009;17(6):361–376.
3. Breitbart W, Lederberg MS, Rueda-Lara M, Alici Y. Psycho-oncology. In: Sadock BJ, Sadock VA, eds. *Kaplan and Sadock's Synopsis of Psychiatry*, 10th ed. Philadelphia: Lippincott Williams & Wilkins, 2009:2314–2353.
4. Breitbart W, Alici Y. Agitation and delirium at the end of life: "We couldn't manage him." *JAMA*. 2008;300(24):2898–2910, E1.
5. Breitbart W, Chochinov H, Passik S. Psychiatric symptoms in palliative medicine. In: Doyle D, Hanks G, Cherny N, Calman K, eds. *Oxford Textbook of Palliative Medicine*, 3rd ed. New York: Oxford University Press; 2004:746–771.
6. Portenoy RK, Thaler HT, Kornblith AB, et al. The Memorial Symptom Assessment Scale: an instrument for the evaluation of symptom prevalence, characteristics, and distress. *Eur J Cancer*. 1994;30A:1326–1336.

Chapter 4

Anxiety Disorders in Palliative Care

Anxiety is common in palliative care patients. It can be a natural response to impending death, uncertainty, and suffering. It may also represent a clinically significant issue adversely affecting patients' quality of life.

Prevalence of Anxiety

The prevalence of anxiety in patients receiving palliative care increases with advancing disease and decline in the patient's physical status.[1,2] In cancer patients, anxiety is commonly associated with depressive symptoms.[1,2] In HIV-positive patients, especially in those who are newly diagnosed, anxiety is most commonly associated with adjustment disorders.[3] Anxiety in palliative care settings can also represent reactivation of a pre-existing anxiety disorder, such as panic disorder or generalized anxiety disorder (Table 4.1).[1]

Anxiety can have many etiologies in the terminally ill population. Situational, psychiatric, organic, and existential types of anxiety have been described in cancer patients based on the main etiological factors underlying anxiety symptoms.[5] Anxiety may be a part of one of the psychiatric disorders, may be a component of pain, dyspnea, and nausea, may be related to medication adverse effects, alcohol or drug withdrawal, or may be related to metabolic causes such as hyperthyroidism.[6–10] Existential concerns about dying, psychosocial concerns about family, and finances could also manifest as anxiety (Table 4.2; Box 4.1).[9]

The terminally ill patient often presents with a complex mixture of physical and psychological symptoms in the context of a frightening reality. Thus, the recognition of anxious symptoms requiring treatment can be challenging (Box 4.2).

Table 4.1 Prevalence of Anxiety Disorders in Palliative Care[1–4]

Patient Population	Prevalence
Advanced melanoma patients	28%
Patients with advanced cancer and AIDS*	10%–28%
Congestive heart failure	50%
Chronic obstructive pulmonary disease	

*Research study findings have often differed with regard to time since notification, stage of disease, gender, and sexual orientation.

Table 4.2 Common Types and Causes of Anxiety in Terminally Ill Patients[6–10]

Types of Anxiety	Causes
Reactive anxiety/adjustment disorder	Awareness of terminal condition
	Fears and uncertainty about death
	Conflicts with family or staff
	End-of-life decision discussions
Disease- and treatment-related anxiety	Poor symptom control (fatigue, depression, nausea, insomnia, dyspnea)
	Poor pain control
	Related metabolic disturbances
	Hypoxia
	Delirium
	Sepsis
	Bleeding
	Pulmonary embolus
Substance-induced anxiety	
Anxiety-producing drugs	Glucocorticosteroids:
	Dexamethasone
	Prednisone
	Antiemetics with dopamine blocking effects: Metoclopramide
	Prochlorperazine
	Bronchodilators
Withdrawal	Opioids
	Benzodiazepines
	Alcohol
	Nicotine
Pre-existing anxiety disorders (generalized anxiety disorder, panic disorder, phobias, posttraumatic stress disorder, adjustment disorder)	Exacerbation of symptoms related to fears and distressing medical symptoms

Box 4.1 Withdrawal States and Anxiety

- During the terminal phase of illness, when patients become less alert, there is a tendency to minimize the use of sedating medications. It is important to consider the need to slowly taper benzodiazepines and opioid analgesics in order to prevent acute withdrawal states.
- Withdrawal states in terminally ill patients often present first as agitation, restlessness, or anxiety.
- Because of impaired metabolism, withdrawal states become clinically evident days later than might be expected in younger, healthier patients.

Box 4.2 Recognizing Symptoms of Anxiety[6,8,9]

- Physical symptoms are the most common presenting symptoms of anxiety in patients with advanced illness.
- The physical or somatic manifestations of anxiety, such as autonomic hyperactivity, insomnia, or dyspnea, often overshadow the psychological or cognitive ones.
- The assumption that a high level of anxiety is inevitably encountered during the terminal phase of illness is neither helpful nor accurate for diagnostic and treatment purposes.

Assessment should include a thorough history and physical examination, including a history of psychiatric disorders, and substance use disorders (e.g., illicit drugs, alcohol). Home-based palliative care patients and palliative care inpatients experience similar rates of anxiety; therefore, palliative care patients in all settings should be screened and assessed for anxiety.[11] Symptoms of anxiety should be differentiated from delirium or akathisia.

The Memorial Symptom Assessment Scale, the Edmonton Symptom Assessment Scale, and the Hospital Anxiety and Depression Scale have been used in clinical settings for screening and assessment of anxiety in palliative care patients.[12–16] The Hospital Anxiety and Depression Scale has been shown to demonstrate highest scores on psychometric properties in a review of outcome measures used in randomized controlled trials of interventions in cancer.[12]

Despite the fact that anxiety in terminal illness commonly results from medical complications, it is important not to forget that psychological factors related to death and dying or existential issues play a role in anxiety, particularly in patients who are alert and not confused.[6] It is the role of the psycho-oncologist to elicit these concerns and listen empathically to them.

When anxiety is severe or distressing drug therapy is considered in addition to supportive care (Box 4.3).

The pharmacotherapy of anxiety in terminal illness involves the judicious use of the following classes of medications: benzodiazepines, typical and atypical antipsychotics, antihistamines, antidepressants, and opioid analgesics.[1,6,8,9,17] A recent Cochrane review was unable to identify any well-designed prospective randomized controlled trials involving the use of drug therapy for the treatment of symptoms of anxiety in adult palliative care patients.[18] Although the

Box 4.3 Treatment of Anxiety in the Terminally Ill[1,6,8,9]

- The treatment is initiated based on the patient's subjective level of distress.
- Consider the risks and benefits of treatment.
- The specific treatment of anxiety in the terminally ill often depends on etiology, presentation, and setting.
- Other considerations include problematic patient behavior such as noncompliance because of anxiety, and family and staff reactions to the patient's distress.

clinical evidence is supportive of the use of the listed medications in the treatment of anxiety among palliative care patients, randomized controlled trials are required to establish the risks and benefits of medication use for this patient population (Table 4.3).

Benzodiazepines are the mainstay of the pharmacological treatment of anxiety in the terminally ill patient. Benzodiazepines are commonly used in palliative care settings for anxiety and other distressing symptoms such as nausea and insomnia.[1,20] It is important to monitor for worsening confusion, fatigue, or

Table 4.3 Medications Used in the Treatment of Anxiety among Patients with Advanced Disease[1,6,8,9,16–18]

	Approximate Daily Dosage Range (mg)	Route*
Benzodiazepines		
Very Short-Acting		
Midazolam	10–60 per 24/h	IV, SC
Short-Acting		
Alprazolam	0.25–2.0 tid-qid	PO, SL
Oxazepam	10–15 tid-qid	PO
Lorazepam	0.5–2.0 tid-qid	PO, SL, IV, IM
Intermediate-Acting		
Chlordiazepoxide	10–50 tid-qid	PO, IM
Long-Acting		
Diazepam	5–10 bid-qid	PO, IM, IV, PR
Clorazepate	7.5–15 bid-qid	PO
Clonazepam	0.5–2 bid-qid	PO
Non-benzodiazepines		
Buspirone	5–20 tid	PO
Typical Antipsychotics		
Haloperidol	0.5–5 q2-12h	PO, IV, SC, IM
Chlorpromazine	12.5-50 q4-12h	PO, IM, IV
Atypical Antipsychotics		
Olanzapine	2.5–20 q12-24h	PO
Risperidone	1–3 q12-24h	PO
Quetiapine fumarate	25–200 q12-24h	PO
Antihistamine		
Hydroxyzine	25–50 q4-6h	PO, IV, SC
Tricyclic Antidepressants		
Imipramine	12.5–150 hs	PO, IM
Clomipramine	10–150 hs	PO

Refer to Table 5.1 in chapter 5 for a list of selective serotonin reuptake inhibitors and serotonin norepinephrine reuptake inhibitors.

* bid, two times a day; IM, intramuscular; IV, intravenous; PO, peroral; PR, per rectum; qid, four times a day; SC, subcutaneous; SL, sublingual; tid, three times a day. Parenteral doses are generally twice as potent as oral doses, intravenous bolus injections or infusions should be administered slowly.

concentration difficulties with the use of benzodiazepines, particularly in older patients (Boxes 4.4 and 4.5).[1]

Antipsychotic medications are considered for the treatment of anxiety when:[1,6,8,9]

1. Benzodiazepines are not sufficient for symptom control.
2. An underlying medical etiology is suspected, particularly for patients at risk for delirium.
3. Psychotic symptoms such as delusions or hallucinations accompany the anxiety.
4. Antipsychotics are perhaps safer when compared with benzodiazepines in patients in whom there is legitimate concern regarding respiratory depression or compromise (Boxes 4.6–4.8).

Box 4.4 Classification and Utilization of Benzodiazepines

Very Short-Acting Benzodiazepine (Midazolam)[19]

- Intravenous infusion is useful in critical care settings in which sedation is the goal in an agitated or anxious patient on a respirator.
- Midazolam seems to be less irritating to subcutaneous tissues than is diazepam, and thus can be given by subcutaneous infusion.
- Because it is several times as potent as diazepam, starting doses should be low, and careful monitoring of effects should be initiated.

Short-Acting Benzodiazepine[8,9]

- The use of shorter-acting benzodiazepines (lorazepam, alprazolam, and oxazepam) is safest in the terminally ill population, avoiding toxic accumulation caused by impaired metabolism in debilitated individuals.
- Lorazepam, oxazepam, and temazepam are metabolized by conjugation (as opposed to oxidative pathways) in the liver and are therefore safest in patients with hepatic disease.
- Dying patients often benefit from parenteral administration of these drugs.
- If patients experience breakthrough anxiety or end of dose failure, consider switching to longer-acting benzodiazepines.

Long-Acting Benzodiazepines[8,9]

- Diazepam can be administered rectally to dying patients when no other route is available (with dosages equivalent to oral regiments). It is useful for the control of anxiety, restlessness, and agitation associated with the final days of life.
- Clonazepam has been found to be extremely useful in the palliative care setting for:
  1. the treatment of anxiety, depersonalization, or derealization in patients with seizure disorders, brain tumors, and mild organic mental disorders
  2. adjuvant analgesia in patients with neuropathic pain
  3. patients who experience end of dose failure with recurrence of anxiety on shorter-acting drugs
  4. tapering off short-acting benzodiazepines

Box 4.5 Utilization of Non-benzodiazepine Anxiolytic (Buspirone)[8,9]

- It is useful in conjunction with psychotherapy for patients with chronic anxiety or anxiety related to adjustment disorders.
- The onset of anxiolytic action is delayed in comparison with the benzodiazepines, taking 5 to 10 days for relief of anxiety to begin.
- It does not prevent or treat benzodiazepine withdrawal. Caution must be used when switching from a benzodiazepine to buspirone.
- Because of its delayed onset of action and indication for use in chronic anxiety states, buspirone may be of limited usefulness to the clinician treating anxiety and agitation in the terminally ill.

Opioid drugs, such as the narcotic analgesics, are primarily indicated for the control of pain.[8,9] Other usages include:[8,9]

1. The relief of dyspnea resulting from cardiopulmonary processes and associated anxiety
2. Continuous intravenous infusions for careful titration and control of respiratory distress, anxiety, pain, and agitation

Box 4.6 Typical and Atypical Antipsychotics

Typical Antipsychotics

- Haloperidol is usually sufficient to control anxiety symptoms and avoid excessive sedation.
- Thioridazine, chlorpromazine, and other lower-potency antipsychotics are effective anxiolytics and can help with insomnia and agitation. They are infrequently used because of concerns for cardiac, anticholinergic, and sedating side effects.
- One must be aware of the potential for extrapyramidal side effects (particularly when patients are taking additional dopamine blocking agents for antiemetic purposes) and the remote possibility of neuroleptic malignant syndrome.
- Tardive dyskinesia is rarely a concern given the generally short-term usage and low dosages of these medications in this population.

Atypical Antipsychotics

- Olanzapine
- Risperidone
- Quetiapine fumarate
- They have anxiolytic properties as typical antipsychotics with lower risk of extrapyramidal side effects or tardive dyskinesia.

Box 4.7 Antihistamine (Hydroxyzine)

- Mild anxiolytic, sedative, and analgesic properties.
- Particularly useful when treating anxious, terminally ill cancer patients with pain.
- Historically, 100 mg given parenterally was found to have analgesic potency equivalent to 8 mg of morphine, and was shown to potentiate the analgesic effects of morphine.[21]
- As an anxiolytic, 25–50 mg of hydroxyzine q 4–6 hours PO, IV, or SC is effective.

Occasionally, one must maintain the patient in a state of unresponsiveness in order to maximize comfort. When respiratory distress is not a major problem, it is preferable to use the opioid drugs solely for analgesic purposes and to add more specific anxiolytics (such as the benzodiazepines) to control concomitant anxiety (Box 4.9).

These interventions may be effective when used alone or in combination. Behavioral interventions have been demonstrated to be quite effective for mild to moderate degrees of anxiety or distress. In highly anxious cancer patients, these techniques should be prescribed concurrently with pharmacological treatment for greater effectiveness and more rapid onset of beneficial action.

For further information on psychotherapeutic and behavioral interventions in the dying patient, see chapter 9.

Box 4.8 Antidepressants[1,6,8,9]

- Selective serotonin reuptake inhibitors (SSRIs) and serotonin norepinephrine reuptake inhibitors are considered to be first-line antidepressants in the treatment of anxiety disorders. However, the delayed onset of action with these medications frequently poses a challenge in terminally ill patients with anxiety symptoms. Drugs that require a period of weeks to achieve therapeutic effect may be unsatisfactory.
- This is the most effective treatment for anxiety accompanying depression and the treatment of panic disorder.
- The usefulness of tricyclic antidepressants (TCAs) is often limited in the dying patient because of anticholinergic and sedative side effects.
- Mirtazapine also has been used to treat anxiety, especially in patients with insomnia and anorexia.
- Older patients are generally more sensitive to anticholinergic effects of TCAs and emetic effects of SSRIs.
- For further guidelines on usage, see the following section on depression.

Box 4.9 Nonpharmacological Interventions for Anxiety and Distress[22–31]

1. Brief supportive psychotherapy is often useful in dealing with both crisis-related issues as well as existential issues confronted by the terminally ill.
2. Behavioral interventions (relaxation, guided imagery)
3. Cognitive behavioral psychotherapy
4. Psychoeducation
5. Hypnosis
6. Massage therapy

References

1. Traeger L. Evidence-based treatment of anxiety in patients with cancer. *J Clin Oncol*, 2012;30(11):1197.
2. Kolva E, Rosenfeld B, Pessin H, Breitbart W, Brescia R. Anxiety in terminally ill cancer patients. *J Pain Symptom Manage*. 2011;42(5):691–701.
3. Kerrihard T, Breitbart W, Dent K, Strout D. Anxiety in patients with cancer and human immunodeficiency virus. *Seminars in Clinical Neuropsychiatry*. 1999;4:114–132
4. Mitchell AJ. Prevalence of depression, anxiety, and adjustment disorder in oncological, haematological, and palliative-care settings: a meta-analysis of 94 interview-based studies. *Lancet Oncol*. 2011;12(2):160.
5. Stiefel F, Razavi D. Common psychiatric disorders in cancer patients: II. Anxiety and acute confusional states. *Support Care Cancer*. 1994;2:233–237.
6. Stoklosa J, Patterson K, Rosielle D, Arnold RM. Anxiety in palliative care: causes and diagnosis. *J Palliat Med*. 2011;14(10):1173–1174.
7. Delgado-Guay M, Parsons HA, Li Z, et al. Symptom distress in advanced cancer patients with anxiety and depression in the palliative care setting. *Support Care Cancer*. 2009;17:573–579.
8. Roth AJ, Massie MJ. Anxiety and its management in advanced cancer. *Curr Opin Support Palliat Care*. 2007;1:50–56.
9. Levin T, Alici Y. Anxiety disorders. In: Holland J, Breitbart W, Jacobsen P, eds. *Psycho-Oncology*, 2nd ed. New York: Oxford University Press, 2010.
10. Brown LF, Kroenke K. Cancer-related fatigue and its associations with depression and anxiety: a systematic review. *Psychosomatics*. 2009;50:440–447.
11. Austin P, Wiley S, McEvoy PM, Archer L. Depression and anxiety in palliative care inpatients compared with those receiving palliative care at home. *Palliat Support Care*. 2011;9(4):393–400.
12. Luckett T, Butow PN, King MT, et al. A review and recommendations for optimal outcome measures of anxiety, depression and general distress in studies evaluating psychosocial interventions for English-speaking adults with heterogeneous cancer diagnoses. *Support Care Cancer*. 2010;18:1241–1262.
13. Bruera E, Kuehn N, Miller MJ, Selmser P, Macmillan K. The Edmonton Symptom Assessment System (ESAS): a simple method of the assessment of palliative care patients. *J Palliat Care* 1991;7:6–9.

14. Zigmond AS, Snaith RP. The hospital anxiety and depression scale. *Acta Psychiatr Scand*. 1983;67:361–370.
15. Portenoy RK, Thaler HT, Kornblith AB, Thaler HT, Kornblith AB, Lepore JM, et al. The Memorial Symptom Assessment Scale: an instrument for the evaluation of symptom prevalence, characteristics and distress. *Eur J Cancer* 1994;30A:1326–1336.
16. Block SD. Psychological issues in end-of-life care. *J Palliat Med*. 2006;9:751–772.
17. Jacobsen PB, Donovan KA, Swaine ZN, et al. Management of anxiety and depression in adult cancer patients: toward an evidence-based approach. In: Chang AE, Ganz PA, Hayes DF, et al., eds. *Oncology: An Evidence-Based Approach*. New York: Springer-Verlag; 2006:1552–1579.
18. Candy B, Jackson KC, Jones L, Tookman A, King M. Drug therapy for symptoms associated with anxiety in adult palliative care patients. *Cochrane Database Syst Rev*. 2012;10:CD004596.
19. Mendoza R, Djenderedjian AH, Adams J, Ananth J. Midazolam in acute psychotic patients with hyperarousal. *J Clin Psychiatry* 1987;48:291–292.
20. Holland JC, Hughes MK, Greenberg DB, eds. *Quick Reference for Oncology Clinicians: The Psychiatric and Psychological Dimensions of Cancer Symptom Management*. Charlottesville, VA: American Psychosocial Oncology Society; 2006
21. Beaver WT, Feise G. Comparison of the analgesic effects of morphine, hydroxyzine and their combination in patients with post-operative pain. In Bonica JJ, ed. *Advances in Pain Research and Therapy*. New York: Raven; 1976:533–557.
22. Sheard T, Maguire P. The effect of psychological interventions on anxiety and depression in cancer patients: results of two meta-analyses. *Br J Cancer* 1999;80:1770–1780.
23. Newell SA, Sanson-Fisher RW, Savolainen NJ. Systematic review of psychological therapies for cancer patients: overview and recommendations for future research. *J Natl Cancer Inst*. 2002;94:558–584.
24. Osborn RL, Demoncada AC, Feuerstein M. Psychosocial interventions for depression, anxiety, and quality of life in cancer survivors: meta-analyses. *Int J Psychiatry Med*. 2006;36:13–34.
25. Jacobsen PB, Jim HS. Psychosocial interventions for anxiety and depression in adult cancer patients: achievements and challenges. *CA Cancer J Clin*. 2008;58:214–230.
26. Duhamel KN, Mosher CE, Winkel G, et al. Randomized clinical trial of telephone-administered cognitive-behavioral therapy to reduce post-traumatic stress disorder and distress symptoms after hematopoietic stem-cell transplantation. *J Clin Oncol*. 2010;28:3754–3761.
27. Moorey S, Cort E, Kapari M, et al. A cluster randomized controlled trial of cognitive behaviour therapy for common mental disorders in patients with advanced cancer. *Psychol Med*. 2009;39:713–723.
28. Greer JA, Park ER, Prigerson HG, et al. Tailoring cognitive-behavioral therapy to treat anxiety comorbid with advanced cancer. *J Cogn Psychother*. 2010;24:294–313.
29. Devine EC, Westlake SK. The effects of psychoeducational care provided to adults with cancer: meta-analysis of 116 studies. *Oncol Nurs Forum* 1995;22:1369–1381.

30. Plaskota M, Lucas C, Evans R, Cook K, Pizzoferro K, Saini T. A hypnotherapy intervention for the treatment of anxiety in patients with cancer receiving palliative care. *Int J Palliat Nurs*. 2012;18(2):69–75.

31. Falkensteiner M, Mantovan F, Müller I, Them C. The use of massage therapy for reducing pain, anxiety, and depression in oncological palliative care patients: a narrative review of the literature. *ISRN Nurs*. 2011;2011:929868.

Chapter 5

Depression in Palliative Care

Prevalence of Depression in Palliative Care

Depressed mood and sadness can be appropriate responses as the terminally ill patient faces death. These emotions may be manifestations of anticipatory grief over the impending loss of one's life, health, loved ones, and autonomy. Nonetheless, major depressive disorder is a common mental health problem arising in the palliative care setting. It is also important to not regard all depressive symptoms as part of a "normal reaction" to cancer or terminal illness. Depression significantly diminishes quality of life, results in significant existential distress, and complicates symptom control, resulting in more frequent admissions to inpatient care settings.[1] Depressive symptoms are associated with poorer treatment compliance, increased desire for hastened death, and completed suicide in palliative care settings (Box 5.1).[2]

Diagnosis of Depression in Palliative Care

Depression is underdiagnosed and undertreated in the palliative care setting (Boxes 5.2–5.5).[1,6–9]

A critical challenge of diagnosing depression in medically ill patients is the interpretation of physical/somatic symptoms of depression. This is outlined in the DSM-IV-TR criteria for major depressive disorder (Table 5.1).

Box 5.1 Prevalence of Depression in Palliative Care

- Depression is prevalent, but under-recognized, underdiagnosed, and undertreated in palliative care settings.
- Approximately 5% to 20% of patients with advanced cancer meet criteria for major depression even when the most stringent criteria are used.[3]
- An additional 15% to 20% of palliative care patients present with depressive disorders that are less severe but can still be a major source of suffering and despair to patients.[1]
- Prevalence of depression in terminally ill cancer patients is at least three times as common as those found in the general population.[4]
- Range increases with higher levels of disability, advanced illness, and pain.[5]
- Higher rates of depression have been reported in patients with pancreatic, gastric, lung, and oropharyngeal cancers.[4]

Box 5.2 Factors Contributing to Underdiagnosis and Undertreatment of Depression in Those with Advanced Illness[1,9]

- Minimization of symptoms and significance of depression by clinicians
- The belief that depression is a completely appropriate reaction among terminally ill cancer patients
- Concern that severely medically ill patients will not be able to tolerate side effects or drug interactions associated with the initiation of antidepressant therapy
- Difficulty of accurately diagnosing depression in the terminally ill

Box 5.3 Risk Factors Associated with Depression in Patients with Advanced Disease[4,10–15]

- Patients with certain types of cancers, such as pancreatic cancer, are more likely to develop depression than patients with other types of intra-abdominal malignancies.
- Family history of depression
- History of previous depressive episodes
- Poor social support
- Poor communication with health care professionals
- The number and severity of physical symptoms
- Studies have found a correlation among depression, pain, and functional status.
- Low scores on measures of spiritual well-being. This highlights the significance of the relationship between existential distress and depression in terminal illness.
- Certain medications and physical conditions may predispose to depression, and should be addressed before initiation of treatment for depression.

Box 5.4 Medications and Physical Conditions Associated with Depression in the Palliative Care Setting[1,11,16–19]

- Corticosteroids
- Chemotherapeutic agents: vincristine, vinblastine, asparaginase, intrathecal methotrexate, interferon, interleukin
- Amphotericin
- Whole brain radiation
- Tumors that originate in or metastasize to the central nervous system
- Central nervous system metabolic-endocrine complications
- Paraneoplastic syndromes

Box 5.5 Five Approaches to the Diagnosis of Major Depression in Patients with Advanced Illness[1,9]

1. *Inclusive approach*: includes all symptoms, whether or not they are secondary to advanced illness or treatment
2. *Exclusive approach*: deletes and disregards all physical symptoms from consideration, not allowing them to contribute to the diagnosis
3. *Etiological approach*: the clinician attempts to determine if the physical symptom is caused by illness or treatment or a depressive disorder
4. *Substitutive approach*: physical symptoms of uncertain etiology are replaced by other nonsomatic symptoms[20]
5. *High-threshold approach*: requires a higher threshold number (7 rather than 5) of diagnostic criteria symptoms to make a diagnosis[21]

Chochinov et al., using the low threshold approach, found that Endicott substitutions identified fewer cases of major depression. However, when using the high-threshold approach, results suggest that the research diagnostic criteria (RDC) and Endicott criteria were equivalent in diagnosis of major depression whether or not one included somatic symptoms. Although researchers have raised concerns regarding the nonspecificity of somatic symptoms in the medically ill, their inclusion may not overly influence the diagnostic classification of major depression.[21]

Table 5.1 DSM-IV Criteria for Major Depressive Disorder and Endicott Substitute Symptoms

DSM-IV Criteria	Endicott Substitute Symptoms
Depressed mood most of the day*	
Markedly diminished interest or pleasure in all or almost all activities most of the day*	
Weight loss/gain; appetite increase/decrease	Depressed appearance; tearfulness
Insomnia or hypersomnia	Social withdrawal; decreased talkativeness
Psychomotor agitation or retardation	
Fatigue or loss of energy	Brooding, self-pity, or pessimism
Feelings of worthlessness or excessive or inappropriate guilt	
Diminished ability to think or concentrate; indecisiveness	Lack of reactivity; cannot be cheered up
Recurrent thoughts of death, suicidal ideation/planning, or a suicide attempt	

* Either depressed mood or diminished interest must be present as one of the five or more symptoms required for a diagnosis of major depression.

The diagnostic interview remains the most commonly used clinical tool, and should directly assess commonly accepted criteria in addition to relying more heavily on the psychological or cognitive symptoms of major depression.[22,23] How is the clinician to interpret feelings of hopelessness in the dying patient when there is no hope for cure or recovery? Feelings of hopelessness, worthlessness, or suicidal ideation must be explored in detail. Although many dying patients lose hope of a cure, they are able to maintain hope for better symptom control. For many patients hope is contingent on the ability to find continued meaning in their day-to-day existence. Hopelessness that is pervasive and accompanied by a sense of despair or despondency is more likely to represent a symptom of a depressive disorder.

Similarly, patients often state that they feel they are burdening their families, causing them great pain and inconvenience. Those beliefs are less likely to represent a symptom of depression than if the patient feels that his or her life has never had any worth, or that he or she is being punished for evil things the patient has done. Suicidal ideation, even in mild or passive form, is very likely associated with significant degrees of depression in terminally ill cancer patients.[21–23]

Depressed mood and loss of pleasure or interest are also important in assessment of depression in patients with advanced illness.[24,25] Almost all patients with advanced illness experience a certain degree of disengagement from areas of interest. However, a pervasive anhedonia that extends to loss of interest and pleasure in almost all activities merits considerable attention as an important indicator of depression in palliative care settings.[1]

Assessment of Depression in Palliative Care

Numerous assessment methods for depression including diagnostic classification systems, structured interview and screening instruments have been used in research (Box 5.6).

Diagnostic assessments using structured interviews are usually used for research purposes. However, most of these structured interviews are time consuming, which limits their use in palliative care settings. Self-report measures are commonly used to increase the clinician's ability to identify depression in terminally ill cancer patients. Chochinov et al. studied brief screening instruments to measure depression in the terminally ill.[26] His group compared the performance of four brief screening measures for depression in a group of terminally ill patients. The single-item interview method (see Box 5.8) correctly identified the diagnosis of every patient, while not misidentifying any patient, substantially outperforming the questionnaire and visual analog measures. Thus, brief screening measures for depression are important clinical tools for terminally ill patients. The performance of the single-item interview, which essentially asks patients if they are depressed, speaks to the importance of mood inquiry in this particularly vulnerable patient population (Box 5.7).

Box 5.6 Assessment Methods for Depression in Patients with Advanced Disease[1]

Diagnostic Classification Systems
Diagnostic and Statistical Manual DSM-III, III-R, IV (1980, 1987, 1994, 2000)
Endicott Substitution Criteria (1984)
Research Diagnostic Criteria (RDC)

Structured Diagnostic Interviews
Schedule for Affective and Schizophrenia (SADS)
Diagnostic Interview Schedule (DIS)
Structured Clinical Interview for DSM-IV (SCID)
Present State Examination (PSE)
Monash Interview for Liaison Psychiatry (MILP)
Mini-International Neuropsychiatric Interview (MINI)
Primary Care Evaluation of Mental Disorders (PRIME-MD)
Structured Interview of Symptoms and Concerns (SISC)

Self-Report Screening Instruments
General Health Questionnaire (GHQ)
Hospital Anxiety and Depression Scale (HADS)
Beck Depression Inventory—Short Form (BDI-SF)
Visual Analog Scale for Depressed Mood
Rotterdam Symptom Checklist (RSCL)
Patient Health Questionnaire-9 (PHQ-9)
Zung Depression Rating Scale

Box 5.7 Single Item Screening Method for Depression in the Terminally Ill[26]

"Have you been depressed most of the day, nearly every day, for the past 2 weeks or more?"

Management of Depression

Depression in cancer patients with advanced disease is optimally managed utilizing a combination of psychotherapy and antidepressant medications.[1,4] Management of depression in advanced cancer patients should include treatment of pain and other distressing physical symptoms along with treatment of depression (Box 5.8).

For further information on psychotherapeutic and behavioral interventions in the dying patient, see chapter 9.

Psychopharmacological Interventions

Use of tricyclic antidepressants (TCAs) in the terminally ill requires a careful risk-benefit ratio analysis (Tables 5.2 and 5.3; Box 5.9).

Box 5.8 Management of Depression in Advanced Cancer Patients[4]

- Psychopharmacological interventions (i.e., antidepressant medications) are the mainstay of management in the treatment of cancer patients with severe depressive symptoms who meet criteria for a major depressive episode.
- The efficacy of antidepressants in the treatment of depression in cancer patients has been well established.[1,23,27–31]
- A variety of psychotherapeutic interventions have been shown to be effective in the treatment of depression and anxiety symptoms related to cancer and cancer pain.[32–40]
- Cognitive behavioral interventions in the form of individual or group psychotherapy have been proved effective in treatment of depressive symptoms in palliative care settings.[1,32]
- Supportive expressive group therapy among advanced breast cancer patients has been shown to ameliorate and prevent new depressive disorders, reduce hopelessness, and improve social functioning.[41]
- Targeted and manualized psychotherapies have been developed, including Meaning-Centered Group Therapy,[42] Dignity Therapy,[43] Mindfulness-Based Meditation Therapy,[44] and a brief supportive-expressive intervention referred to as CALM (Managing Cancer and Living Meaningfully).[45]
- Despite lack of evidence for prolonged survival with a variety of psychosocial interventions, it has been shown through well-designed randomized controlled trials that a variety of psychotherapy interventions are effective in decreasing depressive symptoms and suffering in advanced cancer patients.[46]

Table 5.2 Medications Commonly Used for the Treatment of Depression in Patients with Advanced Illness[1,4]

	Approximate Daily Dosage Range (mg)	Route*
Tricyclic antidepressants		
Amitriptyline	10–150	PO, IM, PR
Desipramine	12.5–150	PO, IM
Nortriptyline	10–125	PO
Doxepin	12.5–150	PO, IM
Imipramine	12.5–150	PO, IM
Clomipramine	10–150	PO
Serotonin-Specific Reuptake Inhibitors (SSRIs)		
Fluoxetine	10–80	PO
Sertraline	25–200	PO
Paroxetine	10–50	PO

(continued)

Table 5.2 (Continued)

	Approximate Daily Dosage Range (mg)	Route*
Citalopram	10–40†	PO
Escitalopram	10–20	PO
Fluvoxamine	50–300	PO
Serotonin-Norepinephrine Reuptake Inhibitor (SNRI)		
Venlafaxine	75–225	PO
Duloxetine	20–60	PO
Serotonin 2 Antagonists/Serotonin Reuptake Inhibitors		
Trazodone	25–300	PO
Nefazodone	100–600	PO
Norepinephrine and Dopamine Reuptake Blockers		
Bupropion	100–450	PO
Bupropion SR‡	100–400	PO
Noradrenergic and Specific Serotonergic Antidepressant		
Mirtazapine	7.5–45	PO
Heterocyclic antidepressants		
Maprotiline	50–75	PO
Amoxapine	100–150	PO
Monoamine oxidase inhibitors		
Isocarboxazid	20–40	PO
Phenelzine	30–60	PO
Tranylcypromine	20–40	PO
Moclobemide	100–600	PO
Benzodiazepines		
Alprazolam	0.25–2.0 tid	PO
Lithium carbonate	150–1200	PO
Psychostimulants		
Dextroamphetamine	2.5–20 bid	PO
Methylphenidate	2.5–20 bid	PO
Modafinil§	50–400¶	PO

* bid, two times a day; IM, intramuscular; PO, peroral; PR, per rectum; tid, three times a day; intravenous infusions of a number of tricyclic antidepressants are utilized outside of the United States. This route is not FDA approved.
† Maximum daily dose is 20 mg for patients >60 years of age.
‡ SR, sustained release
§ This is a wakefulness agent and is not a classic psychostimulant.
¶ Doses >200 mg are rarely more effective.

Box 5.9 Pharmacotherapy for Depression in the Dying Patient: Considerations

- A depressed patient with several months of life expectancy can wait the 2 to 4 weeks it may take to respond to a selective serotonin reuptake inhibitor or a tricyclic antidepressant.
- The depressed dying patient with less than 3 weeks to live may do best with a rapid-acting psychostimulant.[23,47]
- Patients who are within hours to days of death and in distress are likely to benefit most from the use of sedatives or narcotic analgesic infusions for distress relief.

The selective serotonin reuptake inhibitors now have an important role in the pharmacotherapy of depression in the medically ill and those with advanced cancer and AIDS. They have been found to be as effective in the treatment of depression as the tricyclics (Table 5.3; Boxes 5.10 and 5.11).[4]

Side effects of selective serotonin reuptake inhibitors tend to be dose related and may be problematic for patients with advanced disease (Box 5.12).

Psychostimulants are an alternative and effective pharmacologic approach to the treatment of depression in the terminally ill (Boxes 5.13–5.19).[51–53]

In general, monoamine oxidase inhibitors (MAOIs) have been considered a less desirable alternative for treating depression in the terminally ill. They are usually reserved for those who have shown past preferential responses to them for treatment of depression (Boxes 5.20–5.21).

Table 5.3 Medications and Conditions That Exacerbate Tricyclic Antidepressant Side Effects

Sedation	Narcotic analgesics
	Antiemetics
	Anxiolytics
	Neuroleptics
Tachycardia	Cardiac insufficiency
Arrhythmia	Pre-existing conduction defects (especially second- or third-degree heart block)
Postural hypotension and dizziness	Volume depletion
Anticholinergic delirium	Pethidine
	Atropine
	Diphenhydramine
	Phenothiazines

Box 5.10 Use of Tricyclic Antidepressants in Terminally Ill Patients[1,4,9]

- Although nearly 70% of patients treated with a TCA for nonpsychotic depression can anticipate a positive response, these medications are associated with a side effect profile that can be particularly troublesome for terminally ill patients (see Table 5.4).
- The tertiary amines (amitriptyline, doxepin, imipramine) have a greater propensity to cause side effects than do secondary amines (nortriptyline, desipramine). The secondary amines are thus often a preferable choice for the terminally ill.

Box 5.11 Considerations, Dosage, and Administration of Tricyclic Antidepressants[1,4,9]

TCA: Factors to Consider

- the nature of the underlying terminal medical condition
- the characteristics of the depressive episode, past responses to antidepressant therapy, and the specific drug side-effect profile
- A side-effect profile that will be least incompatible with the patient's overall medical condition

TCAs: Dosage

- Start at low doses (10–25 mg qhs) and increase in 10- to 25-mg increments every 2 to 4 days, until a therapeutic dose is attained or side effects become a dose-limiting factor.
- Depressed cancer patients often achieve a therapeutic response at significantly lower doses of TCAs (25–125 mg) than are necessary in the physically well (150–300 g).
- Patients with advanced cancer achieve higher serum tricyclic levels at modest doses. Tricyclics with well-established therapeutic plasma levels (desipramine, nortriptyline, amitriptyline, imipramine) should be prescribed to minimize drug toxicity and more carefully guide the process of drug titration.
- Desipramine and nortriptyline are generally better tolerated in this population than amitriptyline or imipramine.
- Tricyclic antidepressants are also used for neuropathic pain.

TCAs: Administration

- Most tricyclics are available as rectal suppositories for patients who are no longer able to take medication orally.
- Outside of the United States, certain tricyclics are available in intravenous and intramuscular formulations.

Table 5.4 Common Side Effects of Tricyclic Antidepressants and Guidelines for Use in the Terminally Ill[1,4,9,48]

Anticholinergic	**Guidelines**
Urinary retention	Use desipramine, nortriptyline
Decreased gastric motility, constipation	
Stomatitis, dry mouth	
Tachycardia	
Arrhythmia	
Blurred vision	
Anticholinergic delirium	Avoid potently anticholinergic antidepressants in patients already receiving other medications with anticholinergic properties
Alpha 1-blockade	
Postural hypotension and dizziness	Use nortriptyline, protriptyline
H1 histamine receptor blockade	
Sedation and drowsiness	Avoid amitriptyline, doxepin (but may be preferred in patients with insomnia)

Box 5.12 Advantages of Selective Serotonin Reuptake Inhibitor Usage in the Terminally Ill[4]

- Low affinity for adrenergic, cholinergic, and histamine receptors, thus accounting for negligible orthostatic hypotension, urinary retention, memory impairment, sedation, or reduced awareness
- No clinically significant alterations in cardiac conduction
- Generally favorable toleration
- Wider margin of safety than the TCAs in the event of an overdose (They do not require therapeutic drug level monitoring.)

Box 5.13 Selective Serotonin Reuptake Inhibitors: Common Side Effects

- Intestinal hypermotility (loose stools, nausea, vomiting)
- Insomnia
- Headaches
- Sweating
- Bruxism
- Sexual dysfunction
- Anxiety, tremor, restlessness, and akathisia (The latter is relatively rare but it can be problematic for terminally ill patients with Parkinson's disease or those on antidopaminergic agents.)
- Fluoxetine can cause a brief period of appetite suppression, usually lasting for a period of several weeks. Transient weight loss may occur, but weight usually returns to baseline level. *The anorectic properties of fluoxetine have not been a limiting factor in the use of this drug in cancer patients.*

Box 5.14 Considerations and Dosage for Selective Serotonin Reuptake Inhibitors[1,4,9]

SSRIs: Considerations

- Fluoxetine and norfluoxetine do not reach a steady state for 5 to 6 weeks, compared with 4 to 14 days for paroxetine, citalopram, escitalopram, fluvoxamine, and sertraline. These differences are important when switching from an SSRI to another antidepressant.
- If a switch to a monamine oxidase inhibitor is required, the washout period for fluoxetine will be at least 5 weeks, given the potential drug interactions between these two agents.
    - Paroxetine, citalopram, escitalopram, fluvoxamine and sertraline, however, require considerably shorter washout periods (10–14 days) under similar circumstances
- Since fluoxetine has entered the market, there have been several reports of significant drug-drug interactions.
- Citalopram and escitalopram appear to be the SSRIs with the least potential for serious drug-drug interactions.
- All SSRIs can inhibit the hepatic isoenzyme P450 2D6, with escitalopram and citalopram being least potent in this regard.
    - This is important with respect to dose/plasma level rations and drug interactions, because the SSRIs are dependent upon hepatic metabolism.
- Paroxetine, and to a somewhat lesser extent fluoxetine, appear to inhibit the hepatic enzymes responsible for their own clearance.
    - Co-administration of these medications with other drugs that are dependent on this enzyme system for their catabolism (e.g., tricyclics, phenothiazines, type IC antiarrhythmics, and quinidine) should be done cautiously.
- Fluvoxamine has been shown in some instances to elevate the blood levels of propranolol and warfarin by as much as twofold, and should not be prescribed together with these agents.
- For the elderly patient with advanced disease, the dose-response curve for sertraline appears to be relatively linear.
    - On the other hand, small dosage increases of paroxetine can result in dramatic elevations in plasma levels.
- Fluvoxamine tends to be somewhat more sedating than the other SSRIs.
- Fluoxetine and paroxetine should be avoided in patients taking tamoxifen because of their strong cytochrome P450 2D6 inhibition.
- Gastrointestinal bleeding and hyponatremia (syndrome of inappropriate antidiuretic hormone secretion) are rare side effects that should be monitored for in patients taking SSRIs.
- Elderly patients are more sensitive to side effects; therefore, small doses and slow increments are recommended in this age group.
- Citalopram maximum daily allowed dose has been reduced to 40 mg daily and to 20 mg daily in patients greater than 60 years of age because of

(continued)

Box 5.14 (Continued)

reports of increased risk of QT prolongation. In the United States the cardiac adverse effect warning has only been released for citalopram, whereas in Canada an increased risk of QT prolongation warning has also been released for escitalopram.

SSRIs: Dosage

- Selective serotonin reuptake inhibitors can generally be started at their minimally effective doses.
- For the terminally ill, therapy should be initiated at approximately half the usual starting dose used in an otherwise healthy patient.
- Given the long half-life of fluoxetine, some patients may only require this drug every second day.
- If patients experience activating effects on SSRIs, they should be given during the day rather than at bedtime.
- Gastrointestinal upset can be reduced by ensuring the patient does not take medication on an empty stomach.

Box 5.15 Serotonin-Norepinephrine Reuptake Inhibitor (Venlafaxine and Duloxetine)

- No significant affinity for muscarinic, histamine, or alpha$_1$-adrenergic receptors
- Some patients may experience a modest sustained increase in blood pressure with venlafaxine, especially at doses above the recommended initiating dose.
- Compared with the SSRIs, its protein binding (<35%) is very low. Thus, few protein binding induced drug interactions are expected.
- Like other antidepressants, venlafaxine and duloxetine should not be used in patients receiving monamine oxidase inhibitors.
- Both venlafaxine and duloxetine have a generally well-tolerated side effect profile.
- Discontinuation symptoms are more commonly seen with venlafaxine than with duloxetine.
- Venlafaxine is the first line choice for those patients receiving tamoxifen because of lack of cytochrome 2D6 inhibition.
- Venlafaxine is commonly used in reducing hot flashes in women receiving chemotherapy or those with tamoxifen-induced menopause.[49]
- Duloxetine has been used for the treatment of diabetic neuropathy and neuropathic pain.[50]
- Dul oxetine is contraindicated in patients with significant liver disease, and monitoring is recommended for risk of hepatic failure.

Box 5.16 Serotonin 2 Antagonists/Serotonin Reuptake Inhibitors[1,4,9]

- Nefazodone:
  - is much less sedating than trazodone, but more likely to cause gastrointestinal activation
  - does not have significant sexual side effects
  - has been discontinued by the marketing drug company in many countries since 2003 because of the rare incidence of hepatotoxicity. The incidence of severe liver damage was reported as approximately 1 in every 250,000 to 300,000 patient-years.
- Trazodone:
  - has an almost negligible anticholinergic profile
  - has considerable affinity for alpha$_1$-adrenoceptors and may thus predispose patients to orthostatic hypotension and its problematic sequelae (i.e., falls, fractures, head injuries)
  - is very sedating. Low doses (25 to 50 mg qhs) can be helpful in the treatment of the depressed cancer patient with insomnia
  - is highly serotonergic and should be considered when the patient requires adjunct analgesic effects in addition to antidepressant effects
  - has little effect on cardiac conduction, but can cause arrhythmias in patients with premorbid cardiac disease
  - has been associated with priapism and should be used with caution in male patients

Box 5.17 Norepinephrine and Dopamine Reuptake Blockers (Bupropion)

- It has not been studied extensively in patients with advanced cancer.
- Consider prescribing it if patients have a poor response to a reasonable trial of other antidepressants.
- It has minimal effects on sexual functioning.
- Patients should be monitored for agitation, anxiety, restlessness, and insomnia during treatment with bupropion.
- It may have a role in the treatment of depressed terminally ill patients with severe fatigue, hypersomnia, and psychomotor retardation, as it has activating effects similar to the stimulant drugs.
- Increased incidence of seizures (dose-dependent, higher risk at doses >300 mg/day) in patients with central nervous system disorders may limit its use in patients with a seizure disorder or brain cancer, or those at increased risk for seizures.
- Bupropion and its sustained release form have been used as an adjunct to smoking cessation interventions, but this usage is generally limited to healthy patients or those with earlier stages of cancer.

Box 5.18 Noradrenergic and Specific Serotonergic Antidepressant (Mirtazapine)[1,4,9]

- It compares favorably with amitriptyline and trazodone (Further studies are needed to compare its clinical efficacy with that of SSRIs.)
- Case series and open label studies have shown mirtazapine to be effective among cancer patients with depressive symptoms.
- It is generally well tolerated by patients with increased sensitivity to gastro-intestinal disturbances.
- It has minimal effect on sexual functioning.
- It has minimal effect on P450 enzymes.
- It improves appetite and results in weight gain, which may be desirable for cancer patients.
- The marked sedative effect of this medication proves quite useful in patients with sleeping difficulties.
- Because of its sedative effects it may not be the first choice antidepressant for patients with fatigue, severe psychomotor retardation, and hypersomnia.

Box 5.19 Heterocyclic Antidepressants[1,4,9]

- The side effect profiles are similar to the TCAs.
- Maprotiline should be avoided in patients with brain tumors and those who are at risk for seizures.
- Amoxapine has mild dopamine blocking activity, and thus may increase the risk of extrapyramidal symptoms and dyskinesias in patients taking other dopamine blockers (e.g., antiemetics).
- Mianserin (not available in North America) is a serotonergic antidepressant with adjuvant analgesic properties that is used widely in Europe and Latin America. It is a safe and effective drug for the treatment of depression in cancer.

Box 5.20 Advantages of Using Psychostimulants

- More rapid onset of action than the SSRIs
- Helpful for patients with dysphoric mood, severe psychomotor slowing, and mild cognitive impairment
- Shown to improve attention, concentration, and overall performance on neuropsychological testing in the medically ill
- In relatively low dose, stimulate appetite, promote a sense of well-being, and improve feelings of weakness and fatigue in cancer patients

Box 5.21 Side Effects of Psychostimulants

- Nervousness and overstimulation
- Mild increase in blood pressure and pulse rate
- When used in palliative care settings, abuse does not appear to be a problem unless the patient has a history of substance abuse or dependence.
- Tremor
- *Rare side effects*:
  1. dyskinesias or motor tics
  2. paranoid psychosis
  3. exacerbation of an underlying and unrecognized confusion state

Box 5.22 Selection of Psychostimulants[51–53]

- Methylphenidate and dextroamphetamine have been shown to reduce sedation secondary to opioid analgesics and provide adjuvant analgesia in cancer patients.
- Modafinil and armodafinil (technically wakefulness agents and not classic psychostimulants) have been approved for use in the United States for the treatment of excessive daytime sleepiness caused by narcolepsy and other medical conditions. Although more controlled studies need to be completed, early case series reports suggest the efficacy of these agents as an antidepressant.

Potential use and benefits include:

1. augmenting agent for treatment-resistant depression, particularly when patients complain of fatigue as one of their symptoms
2. alternative to classic psychostimulants for patients who are unable to tolerate methylphenidate or dextroamphetamine, or for whom these classic psychostimulants are contraindicated
3. low abuse potential
4. less sympathomimetic than the other psychostimulants, with lower potential for adverse cardiovascular effects and seizures

The new, reversible inhibitors of monoamine oxidase-A (RIMAs) have not been studied in the depressed terminally ill, but may eventually have a larger role to play than the nonselective MAOIs. They may reduce some of the problems associated with the older MAOIs (e.g., tranylcypromine, isocarboxazid). However, the RIMAs will likely remain a second-line choice to other available non-MAOI antidepressants (Boxes 5.25–5.27).

Open-label studies of ketamine in physically healthy patients with treatment-resistant depression have found rapid, short-lasting, clinically moderate to large benefits with N-methyl-D-aspartate (NMDA) receptor

Box 5.23 Usage, Dosage, and Administration of Psychostimulants

- Tolerance will develop and adjustment of dose may be necessary
- Treatment with dextroamphetamine or methylphenidate usually begins with a dose of 2.5 mg at 8 a.m. and noon. The dose can be gradually increased over several days until improvement is achieved. Doses are usually less than 20 mg a day, although higher doses may be considered if tolerated by the patient
- Patients are usually maintained on methylphenidate for 1 to 2 months, and approximately two-thirds can discontinue methylphenidate without a recurrence of depressive symptoms. Those who do recur can be maintained on a psychostimulant for up to 1 year without significant abuse problems.
- Occasionally, treatment may be initiated concurrently with an SSRI so that patients with depression may receive the immediate benefits of the psychostimulant drug while the SSRI begins to work. A decision can then be made to either continue without the psychostimulant (if the SSRI has begun to take effect), or to restart and continue treatment with the psychostimulant drug.
- Elderly or frail patients taking modafinil should be started at 50 mg. The dose can then be titrated upward.

Box 5.24 Adverse Interactions, Side Effects, and Contraindications of Monoamine Oxidase Inhibitors[1,4,9]

- Hypertensive crisis, potentially leading to strokes and fatalities may occur with:
  1. Foods rich in tyramine
  2. Sympathomimetic drugs (amphetamines, methylphenidate)
  3. Medications containing phenylpropanolamine and pseudoephedrine
- Concurrent treatment with MAOIs and opioid analgesics has been associated with myoclonus and delirium.[26]
- Meperidine is absolutely contraindicated, as it can lead to hyperpyrexia, cardiovascular collapses and death.
- Monoamine oxidase inhibitors can also cause considerable orthostatic hypotension.

Box 5.25 Reversible Inhibitors of Monoamine Oxidase-A (RIMAs)

- Selectively inhibit MAO-A enzyme, therefore leaving MAO-B enzyme available to deal with any tyramine challenge
- Moclobemide (not available in the United States):
  - does not require dietary restriction of tyramine because of its loose binding to the MAO-A receptor and its short half-life
  - has a far more favorable side effect profile than nonselective MAOIs and tends to be well tolerated
  - still requires avoidance of meperidine, procarbazine, dextromethorphan, or other ephedrine-containing agents
  - requires appropriate dosage adjustments with cimetidine, which increases its plasma concentration

Box 5.26 Lithium Carbonate[1,4,9]

- Patients who have been receiving lithium carbonate before an advanced illness could be maintained on it throughout their treatment.
- Close monitoring is necessary in the preoperative and postoperative periods when fluids and salt may be restricted.
- Maintenance doses of lithium may need reduction in seriously ill patients.
- Lithium should be prescribed with caution for patients receiving cis-platinum because of the potential nephrotoxicity of both drugs.

Box 5.27 Benzodiazepines[1]

- Benzodiazepines are not antidepressants.
- Alprazolam has been shown to be a mildly effective antidepressant as well as an anxiolytic. It is particularly useful in cancer patients who have mixed symptoms of anxiety and depression.
- Improvement in depressive symptoms with benzodiazepines is likely secondary to their anxiolytic properties. There is no substantial evidence of benefit for depression from treatment with benzodiazepines alone.

antagonists, such as ketamine, although the long-term benefits and risks are unknown.[54–59] Case reports also suggest that ketamine can rapidly improve depressive symptoms in patients with refractory depression in the setting of a terminal illness.[54–59] However, the optimal selection of patients for this approach and the best way in which to administer ketamine in this situation are unclear.

Occasionally, it is necessary to consider electroconvulsive therapy (ECT) for depressed patients with advanced illness who have depression with psychotic features, depression with catatonic features, or in whom treatment with antidepressants poses unacceptable side effects. The safe and effective use of ECT in the medically ill has been reviewed by others.[1]

References

1. Wilson K, Lander M, Chochinov HM. Diagnosis and management of depression in palliative care. In: Chochinov H, Breitbart W, eds. *Handbook of Psychiatry in Palliative Medicine*. New York: Oxford University Press, 2009:39–68.
2. Li M, Boquiren V, Lo C, et al. Depression and anxiety in supportive oncology. In: Davis M, Feyer P, Ortner P, et al., eds. *Supportive Oncology*. Philadelphia: Elsevier; 2011:528–540.
3. Wilson KG, Chochinov HM, Skirko MG, Allard P, Chary S, Gagnon PR, et al. Depression and anxiety disorders in palliative cancer care. *J Pain Symptom Manage*. 2007a;33(2):118–129.
4. Li M, Fitzgerald P, Rodin G. Evidence-based treatment of depression in patients with cancer. *JCO* 2012;1187–1196.
5. Weinberger MI, Whitbourne SK. Depressive symptoms, self-reported physical functioning, and identity in community-dwelling older adults. *Ageing* Int. 2010;35(4):276–285.

6. Lloyd-Williams M, Friedman T, Rudd N. A survey of antidepressant prescribing in the terminally ill. *J Palliat Med*. 1999;13:243–248.
7. Sharpe M, Strong V, Allen K, Rush R, Tulloh A, Maguire P, et al. Major depression in outpatients attending a regional cancer centre: screening and unmet treatment needs. *Br J Cancer* 2004;90:314–320.
8. Bruera E, Kuehn N, Miller MJ, Selmser P, Macmillan K. The Edmonton Symptom Assessment System (ESAS): a simple method for the assessment of palliative care patients. *J Palliat Care* 1991;(7):6–9.
9. Miller K, Massie MJ. Depressive disorders. In: Holland J, Breitbart W, Jacobsen P, eds. *Psycho-Oncology*, 2nd ed. New York: Oxford University Press, 2010.
10. Li M, Rodin G. Depression. In: Levenson JL, ed. *Textbook of Psychosomatic Medicine: Psychiatric Care of the Medically Ill*, 2nd ed. Arlington, VA: American Psychiatric Publishing; 2011:175–197.
11. Holland JC, Korzun AH, Tross S, Silberfarb P, Perry M, Comis R, et al. Comparative psychological disturbance in patients with pancreatic and gastric cancer. *Am J Psychiatry* 1986;143:982–986.
12. Clark KL, Loscalzo M, Trask PC, et al. Psychological distress in patients with pancreatic cancer: an understudied group. *Psychooncology* 2010;19:1313–1320.
13. Li M, Boquiren V, Lo C, et al. Depression and anxiety in supportive oncology. In: Davis M, Feyer P, Ortner P, et al. eds. *Supportive Oncology*. Philadelphia: Elsevier; 2011:528–540.
14. Rodin G, Zimmermann C, Rydall A, et al. The desire for hastened death in patients with metastatic cancer. *J Pain Symptom Manage*. 2007;33:661–675.
15. Nelson CJ, Rosenfeld B, Breitbart W, Galietta M. Spirituality, religion, and depression in the terminally ill. *Psychosomatics* 2002;43:213–220.
16. Brown JH, et al. Cancer and depression. Cancer presenting with depressive illness: an autoimmune disease? *Br J Psychiatry* 1982:141;227–232.
17. Massie MJ, et al. Depression and suicide in patients with cancer. *J Pain Symptom Manage*. 1994;9:325–340.
18. Lynch ME. The assessment and prevalence of affective disorders in advanced cancer. *J Palliat Care* 1995;11:10–18.
19. Breitbart W. Psychiatric management of cancer pain. *Cancer* 1989;63:2336–2342.
20. Endicott J. Measurement of depression in patients with cancer. *Cancer* 1984;53:2243–2249.
21. Chochinov HM, Wilson KG, Enns M, Lander S. Prevalence of depression in the terminally ill: effects of diagnostic criteria and symptom threshold judgments. *Am J Psychiatry* 1994;151:537–540.
22. Kathol RG, Mutgi A, Williams J, Clamon G, Noyes R. Diagnosis of major depression in cancer patients according to four sets of criteria. *Am J Psychiatry* 1990;147:1021–1024.
23. Block SD. Assessing and managing depression in the terminally ill patient. *Ann Intern Med*. 2000;132:209–218.
24. Spoletini I, Gianni W, Repetto L, Bria P, Caltagirone C, Bossù P, et al. Depression and cancer: an unexplored and unresolved emergent issue in elderly patients. *Crit Rev Oncol Hematol*. 2008;65(2):143–155.
25. Weinberger MI, Roth AJ, Nelson CJ. Untangling the complexities of depression diagnosis in older cancer patients. *Oncologist* 2009;14(1):60–66.
26. Chochinov HM, Wilson KG, Enns M, Lander S. "Are you depressed?" Screening for depression in the terminally ill. *Am J Psychiatry* 1997;154:674–676.

27. Jacobsen PB, Donovan KA, Swaine ZN, et al. Management of anxiety and depression in adult cancer patients: toward an evidence-based approach. In: Chang AE, Ganz PA, Hayes F, et al., eds. *Oncology: An Evidence-Based Approach.* New York: Springer-Verlag; 2006:1552–1579.
28. Williams S, Dale J. The effectiveness of treatment for depression/depressive symptoms in adults with cancer: a systematic review. *Br J Cancer* 2006;94:372–390.
29. Rodin G, Lloyd N, Katz M, et al. The treatment of depression in cancer patients: a systematic review. *Support Care Cancer* 2007;15:123–136.
30. Ng CG, Boks MP, Zainal NZ, et al. The prevalence and pharmacotherapy of depression in cancer patients. *J Affect Disord.* 2011;131:1–7.
31. Rayner L, Price A, Evans A, et al. Antidepressants for the treatment of depression in palliative care: systematic review and meta-analysis. *Palliat Med.* 2011;25:36–51.
32. Spiegel D, Bloom JR, Yalom I. Group support for patients with metastatic cancer. A randomized outcome study. *Arch Gen Psychiatry* 1981;38:527–533
33. Holland JC, Morrow GR, Schmale A, Derogatis L, Stefanek M, Brenson S, et al. Randomized clinical trial of alprazolam versus progressive muscle relaxation in cancer patients with anxiety and depressive symptoms. *J Clin Oncol.* 1991;9:1004–1011.
34. Liossi C, White P. Efficacy of clinical hypnosis in the enhancement of quality of life of terminally ill cancer patients. *Contemp Hypn.* 2001;18:145–160.
35. Kissane DW, Grabsch B, Clarke DM, et al. Supportive-expressive group therapy for women with metastatic breast cancer: survival and psychosocial outcome from a randomized controlled trial. *Psychooncology* 2007;16:277–286.
36. Edelman S, Bell DR, Kidman AD. A group cognitive behaviour therapy programme with metastatic breast cancer patients. *Psychooncology* 1999;8:295–305.
37. Goodwin PJ, Leszcz M, Ennis M, et al. The effect of group psychosocial support on survival in metastatic breast cancer. *N Engl J Med* 2001;345:1719–1726.
38. Classen C, Butler LD, Koopman C. Supportive-expressive group therapy and distress in patients with metastatic breast cancer: a randomized clinical intervention trial. *Arch Gen Psychiatry* 2001;58:494–501.
39. Savard J, Simard S, Giguere I, et al. Randomised clinical trial on cognitive therapy for depression in women with metastatic breast cancer: psychological and immunological effects. *Palliat Support Care* 2006;4:219–237.
40. Breitbart W, Rosenfeld B, Gibson C, et al. Meaning-centered group psychotherapy for patients with advanced cancer: a pilot randomized controlled trial. *Psychooncology* 2010;19:21–28.
41. Kissane DW, Grabsch B, Clarke DM, Smith GC, Love AW, Bloch S, et al. Supportive-expressive group therapy for women with metastatic breast cancer: survival and psychosocial outcome from a randomized controlled trial. *Psychooncology* 2007a;16(4):277–286.
42. Breitbart W, Rosenfeld B, Gibson C, Pessin H, Poppito S, Nelson C, et al. Meaning-centered group psychotherapy for patients with advanced cancer: a pilot randomized controlled trial. *Psycho-oncology* 2010(1):21–28.
43. Chochinov HM, Hack T, Hassard T, et al. Dignity therapy: a novel psychotherapeutic intervention for patients near the end of life. *J Clin Oncol* 2005;23:5520–5525.
44. Ando MT, Morita T, Akechi T, et al. The efficacy of mindfulness-based meditation therapy on anxiety, depression, and spirituality in Japanese patients with cancer. *J Palliat Med* 2009;12:1091–1094.

45. Nissim R, Freeman E, Lo C, et al. Managing Cancer and Living Meaningfully (CALM): A qualitative study of a brief individual psychotherapy for individuals with advanced cancer. *Palliat Med* [epub ahead of print October 31, 2011]

46. Kissane DW. Letting go of the hope that psychotherapy prolongs cancer survival. *JCO* 2007b:5689–5690.

47. Homsi J, Nelson KA, Sarhill N, Rybicki L, LeGrand SB, Davis MP, et al. A phase II study of methylphenidate for depression in advanced cancer. *Am J Hospice Palliat Care* 2001;18:403–417.

48. Preskorn SH, Jerkovich GS. Central nervous system toxicity of tricyclic antidepressants: phenomenology, course, risk factors, and role of therapeutic drug monitoring. *J Clin Psychopharmacol.* 1990;10:88–95.

49. Loprinzi CL, Kugler JW, Sloan JA, et al. Venlafaxine in management of hot flashes in survivors of breast cancer: a randomised controlled trial. *Lancet* 2000;356:2059–2063.

50. Jann MW, Slade JH. Antidepressant agents for the treatment of chronic pain and depression. *Pharmacotherapy* 2007;27:1571–1578.

51. Abbasowa L, Kessing LV, Vinberg M, Nord J. Psychostimulants in moderate to severe affective disorder: a systematic review of randomized controlled trials. *Psychiatry* January 7, 2013 [Epub ahead of print].

52. Calabrese JR, Ketter TA, Youakim JM, Tiller JM, Yang R, Frye MA. Adjunctive armodafinil for major depressive episodes associated with bipolar I disorder: a randomized, multicenter, double-blind, placebo-controlled, proof-of-concept study. *J Clin Psychiatry* 2010;71(10):1363–1370.

53. Menza MA, Kaufmann KR, Castellanos A. Modafinil augmentation of antidepressant treatment in depression. *J Clin Psychiatry* 2000;61:378–381.

54. Zanicotti CG, Perez D, Glue P. Mood and pain responses to repeat dose intramuscular ketamine in a depressed patient with advanced cancer. *J Palliat Med.* 2012;15:400.

55. Stefanczyk-Sapieha L, Oneschuk D, Demas M. Intravenous ketamine "burst" for refractory depression in a patient with advanced cancer. *J Palliat Med.* 2008;11:1268.

56. Yang C, Zhou ZQ, Yang JJ. Be prudent of ketamine in treating resistant depression in patients with cancer. *J Palliat Med.* 2011;14:537.

57. Thangathurai D, Roby J, Roffey P. Treatment of resistant depression in patients with cancer with low doses of ketamine and desipramine. *J Palliat Med.* 2010;13:235.

58. Kollmar R, Markovic K, Thürauf N, et al. Ketamine followed by memantine for the treatment of major depression. *Aust N Z J Psychiatry* 2008;42:170.

59. Irwin SA, Iglewicz A. Oral ketamine for the rapid treatment of depression and anxiety in patients receiving hospice care. *J Palliat Med.* 2010;13:903.

Chapter 6

Suicide, Assisted Suicide, and Desire for Hastened Death

Suicide, suicidal ideation, and desire for hastened death are all important and serious consequences of unrecognized and inadequately treated clinical depression. Although clinical depression is a critically important factor in desire for hastened death, it is not the only reason patients with a terminal illness wish or seek to hasten their death. Desire for hastened death is one the most controversial topics in palliative care. Despite legal prohibitions against assisted suicide, a substantial number of patients think about and discuss those alternatives with their physicians, family, and friends.[1] Those alternatives may range from passive death wishes, contemplating suicide, or requesting the physicians' aid in dying sooner. Although several studies have explored suicide, suicidal ideation, and the desire for hastened death in the terminally ill, questions remain around the prevalence, assessment, and management of these phenomena (Table 6.1).[1]

Cancer patients are at increased risk of suicide relative to the general population, particularly in the terminal stage of illness. Despite the increased risk of suicide among terminally ill patients, the prevalence of completed suicide attempts in patients with terminal illness has not been studied extensively. In a study from Norway examining the completed suicide data from the Cancer Registry of Norway standard mortality ratios of 1.55 for males and 1.35 for females were identified, respectively.[6] However, it is rare for a cancer patient to commit suicide without some degree of premorbid psychopathology that places him or her at increased risk.[1] Cancer patients most frequently commit suicide in the advanced stages of disease (Table 6.2).[1]

It is notable that the completed assisted suicides are rare. Assisted suicides account for 0.2% of all the deaths (including people who were not terminally ill, such as deaths caused by accidents) in Oregon or about 1/500 Oregonians who

Table 6.1 Prevalence of Suicidal Ideation and Desire for Hastened Death (DHD) in Patients with Advanced Illness

Patient Population	Prevalence of Suicidal Ideation and DHD
185 cancer patients with pain studied at MSKCC[*,2]	17%
92 terminally ill patients[†,3]	17%
379 patients with terminal cancer[†,4]	39.8%
200 terminally ill patients in a palliative care facility[5]	44.5% (fleeting)
	8.5% (sustained)

* Memorial Sloan Kettering Cancer Center.
† Desire for hastened death.

Table 6.2 Interest in Physician-Assisted Suicide among Patients with Advanced Illness

Patient Population	
Terminally ill AIDS patients[7]	55%
Advanced cancer patients[8]	25% seriously considered
	12% discussed with physician

die each year.[9] These findings are supportive of the fact that most terminally ill patients want to talk about their options, but very few ultimately need a medically assisted death even in an environment in which it is legally permissible. Physician-assisted suicide is legal in the Netherlands, Belgium, and Switzerland, and in the States of Oregon, Washington, and Montana in the United States.[10] Regardless of the legalization of physician-assisted suicide, the primary goal of the clinician should be to assess the complexity of each case individually with particular attention to underlying depression, hopelessness, and physical distress when faced with these requests (Table 6.3; Boxes 6.1–6.4).[11]

Table 6.3 Estimated Prevalence of Psychiatric Disorders in Suicidal Cancer Patients[1]

Major depression	33%
Delirium	20%
Adjustment disorder with both anxious and depressed features	50%
Personality disorders	50%

Box 6.1 Factors Associated with Increased Risk of Suicide and Desire for Hastened Death in Patients with Advanced Disease[1,4,12]

1. Pain or other physical suffering
2. Advanced illness with a poor prognosis
3. Depression—particularly with feelings of hopelessness
4. Disinhibition resulting from delirium
5. Loss of control* and feelings of helplessness
6. Loss of autonomy
7. Existential distress in the form of loss of meaning, loss of purpose, loss of dignity, and/or awareness of incomplete tasks
8. Physical impairment (see Box 6.2)
9. Pre-existing psychopathology
10. Substance/alcohol abuse
11. Family history of a psychiatric illness and suicide
12. Personal history of a psychiatric illness and suicide
13. Emotional or physical fatigue and exhaustion
14. Lack of social support or social isolation (see Box 6.3)

*"Loss of control" refers to both the helplessness induced by physical symptoms or deficits, as well as the inability to control one's environment.

Box 6.2 Important Physical Impairment Factors in Patients with Suicidal Ideation and Desire for Hastened Death among the Terminally Ill[1,4]

1. Delirium or other forms of cognitive impairment
2. Loss of mobility
3. Paraplegia
4. Loss of bowel and bladder function
5. Amputation
6. Aphonia
7. Sensory loss
8. Inability to eat or swallow
9. Poor functional status

Box 6.3 Important Social Factors in Patients with Suicidal Ideation and Desire for Hastened Death among the Terminally Ill[1,4]

1. Social support
2. Spiritual well-being
3. Quality of life
4. Perception of oneself as a burden to others
5. Loss of meaning

Box 6.4 Depression and Suicide/Desire for Hastened Death in the Dying Patient

- Chochinov et al. found that patients with depression were approximately six to seven times more likely to have a desire for hastened death than patients without depression.[13]
- Breitbart et al. found that patients with a major depression were four times more likely to have a high desire for hastened death.[3] The prevalence of DHD was 47% among patients with depression in comparison to a rate of 12% among patients who were not depressed. *No significant association with the presence or the intensity of pain was found.*[3]
- Van der Lee et al.[14] found that among 138 terminally ill cancer patients, 22% requested assisted suicide. Of the 22% of patients who requested assisted suicide, 23% were depressed at baseline. The rate of request for assisted suicide among patients with depression was 4.1 times greater than that of patients without depression.[14]
- Both depression and hopelessness are unique and synergistic determinants of desire for hastened death.

(continued)

Box 6.4 (Continued)

- Hopelessness is a significantly better predictor of both suicidal ideation and completed suicide than is depression alone.[1,15]
- The 3-, 7-, and 13-item abbreviated version of the Hopelessness Scale have been validated in terminally ill patients, and has been found to overcome the limitations of the original 20-item Hopelessness Scale that is primarily applicable to healthy individuals.[15]
- It is important for clinicians to differentiate expressions of a desire for hastened death from suicidal ideation to address patient concerns and intervene appropriately.[1]
- Severely depressed patients may be more likely than patients with mild or moderate depression to alter their decisions regarding life-sustaining medical treatment once their depression has been treated.[1]

Assessment of suicide risk and appropriate intervention are critical. Early and comprehensive psychiatric involvement with high-risk individuals can often avert suicide in the cancer setting.[1] The myth that asking about suicidal thoughts "puts the idea in their head," is one that should be dispelled, especially in cancer patients. Indeed, patients often reconsider and reject the idea of suicide when the physician acknowledges the legitimacy of their option and the need to retain a sense of control over aspects of their death (Box 6.5).

The response of a clinician to a patient's expression of desire for death or request for assisted suicide has important and obvious implications on all aspects of care that impact on patients, family, and staff.[1] These issues must be addressed both rapidly and thoughtfully (Box 6.6).

Box 6.5 Guidelines for Evaluation of Suicidal Ideation and Desire for Hastened Death in the Terminally Ill[1,16,17]

1. Establish rapport with the patient. Be empathic. Empathic listening skills can be a very therapeutic intervention with the patient in itself.[18] Do not appear critical or state that the patient's thoughts are inappropriate. Be nonjudgmental. Convey to the patient that these thoughts are completely acceptable for discussion.
2. Be alert to your own responses as the clinician, be aware of "countertransference" issues and personal fears of death. (Seek supervision, be aware of how your responses influence communication, and monitor your own attitude.)
3. As you elicit the patient's thoughts, explore the meaning of these suicidal thoughts.
4. Explore the seriousness of the risk. Assess history, degree of intent, and quality of internal and external controls. The suicide vulnerability factors listed in Boxes 6.3, 6.4, and 6.5 should be utilized as a guide.
5. Assess relevant mental status.

Box 6.6 Intervention Guidelines for Suicidal Ideation and Desire for Hastened Death in the Terminally Ill[1,16,17,19]

1. Physical and psychological symptoms and syndromes contributing to desire for death should be aggressively treated. Underlying causes such as delirium, pain, lack of social support, feelings of burden, family conflicts, or unrecognized/untreated depression/anxiety should be addressed specifically wherever possible.
2. Initiate a crisis intervention–oriented psychotherapeutic approach, mobilizing as much of the patient's support system as possible. The presence of a strong support system for the patient may act as an external control of suicidal behavior, and significantly reduces risk of suicide in cancer patients.
3. Interventions developed to more specifically address hopelessness and related constructs (e.g., existential concerns, loss of dignity, loss of meaning, demoralization, and spiritual suffering or distress) should be initiated. Several of these specific therapeutic approaches to despair at the end of life are described in detail in chapter 9.
4. Be clear about what is and is not within one's professional mandate (e.g., offer care; eliminate the suffering not the sufferer, obey the law).
5. Psychiatric hospitalization can sometimes be helpful but is usually not desirable in the terminally ill patient.
6. Although it is appropriate to intervene when medical or psychiatric factors are clearly the driving force in a cancer suicide attempt, there are circumstances in which usurping control from the patient and family with overly aggressive intervention may be less helpful. This is most evident in those with advanced illness, in whom comfort and symptom control are the primary concerns.
7. Summarize and review important points, clarify patient perceptions, provide opportunity for questions, facilitate discussion with others, and provide appropriate referrals.
8. Assure commitment to ongoing care (nonabandonment).

References

1. Olden M, Pessin H, Lichtenthal WG, Breitbart W, et al. Diagnosis and management of depression in palliative care. In: Chochinov H, Breitbart W, eds. *Handbook of Psychiatry in Palliative Medicine*, 2nd ed. New York: 2009:101–112.
2. Breitbart W. Suicide in cancer patients. *Oncology* 1987;1:49–55.
3. Breitbart W, Rosenfeld B, Pessin H, et al. Depression, hopelessness, and desire for hastened death in terminally ill patients with cancer. *JAMA*. 2000;284:2907–2911.
4. Wilson KG, Chochinov HM, McPherson CJ, Skirko MG, Allard P, Chary S, et al. Desire for euthanasia or physician-assisted suicide in palliative cancer care. *Health Psychol*. 2007b;26(3):314–323.
5. Chochinov HMC, Wilson KG, Enns M, Mowchun N, Lander S, Levitt M, et al. Desire for death in the terminally ill. *Am J Psychiatry* 1995;152:1185–1191.
6. Hem E, Loge JH, Haldorsen T, Ekeberg Ø. Suicide risk in cancer patients from 1960 to 1999. *J Clin Oncol*. 2004;22(20):4209–4216.

7. Breitbart W, Rosenfeld B, Passik SD. Interest in physician-assisted suicide among ambulatory HIV-infected patients. *Am J Psychiatry* 1996;153:238–242.
8. Emmanuel EJ, Fairclough DL, Daniels ER, et al. Euthanasia and physician-assisted suicide: attitudes and experiences of oncology patients, oncologists and the public. *Lancet* 1996;347:1805–1810.
9. Quill TE. Physicians should "assist in suicide" when it is appropriate. *J Law Med Ethics* 2012;40(1):57–65.
10. Prokopetz JJ, Lehmann LS. Redefining physicians' role in assisted dying. *N Engl J Med.* 2012;367(2):97–99.
11. Breitbart W. Physician-assisted suicide ruling in Montana: struggling with care of the dying, responsibility, and freedom in Big Sky Country. *Palliat Support Care* 2010;8(1):1–6.
12. Rosenfeld B, Breitbart W, Gibson C, Kramer M, Tomarken A, Nelson C, et al. Desire for hastened death among patients with advanced AIDS. *Psychosomatics* 2006;47(6):504–512.
13. Chochinov HMC, Wilson KG, Enns M, Mowchun N, Lander S, Levitt M, et al. Desire for death in the terminally ill. *Am J Psychiatry* 1995;152:1185–1191.
14. van der Lee ML, van der Bom JG, Swarte NB, Heintz AP, de Graeff A, van den Bout J. Euthanasia and depression: a prospective cohort study among terminally ill cancer patients. *J Clin Oncol* 2005 Sep 20;23(27):6607–6612. Epub August 22, 2005.
15. Abbey J, et al. Hopelessness at the end of life: the utility of the hopelessness scale with terminally ill cancer patients. *Br J Health Psychol.* 2005;(10):1–11.
16. Hudson PL, Schofield P, Kelly B, Hudson R, O'Connor M, Kristjanson LJ, et al. Responding to desire to die statements from patients with advanced disease: recommendations for health professionals. *Palliat Med.* 2006;20(7):703–710.
17. National Health and Medical Research Council, Australia. Clinical Practice Guidelines for the Psychosocial Care of Adults with Cancer; 2003.
18. Quill TE. Doctor, I want to die. Will you help me? *JAMA.* 1993;270:870–873.
19. Breitbart W, Rosenfeld B, Gibson C, Kramer M, Li Y, Tomarken A, et al. Impact of treatment for depression on desire for hastened death in patients with advanced AIDS. *Psychosomatics.* 2010b;51(2):98–105. doi: 10.1176/appi.psy.51.2.98.

Chapter 7

Delirium in Palliative Care

Prevalence and Nature of Delirium in Palliative Care

Delirium is the most common and serious neuropsychiatric complication in the patient with advanced cancer.[1,2] Delirium is often under-recognized or misdiagnosed in terminally ill patients. Delirium is highly prevalent in the terminally ill and is a source of morbidity in patients, family members, and staff. Delirium is often a harbinger of impending death and can significantly interfere with pain and symptom control (Table 7.1; Box 7.1).[2–6]

Cognitive impairments of several types (Box 7.2) are common in patients with advanced illness. Although virtually all of these disorders can be seen in the patient with advanced cancer, the most common include delirium and dementia resulting from a general medical condition. It is important to note that patients with mood, anxiety, or psychotic disorders caused by a general medical condition may present with cognitive impairment.[1] Therefore, clinicians should assess for fatigue, poor motivation, depressed mood, severe anxiety, and preoccupation with delusions or hallucinations in palliative care patients who present with cognitive impairment, especially in the absence of a past psychiatric history (Box 7.3).

There have been a number of studies studying delirium-related distress among patients, family caregivers, and health care professionals since publication of the original study summarized in Box 7.4 by Breitbart et al.[3,4–6] More recent studies have supported the findings of that study and set the stage for

Table 7.1 Estimated Prevalence of Delirium in the Medically Ill[1,2,7–9]

Patient Population	Estimated Prevalence
Cancer and AIDS patients with advanced disease	25%–85%
Hospitalized cancer patients seen in psychiatric consultation	25%
Terminal cancer patients	85%
Hematopoietic stem cell transplant patients around the time of transplant	50%
Postoperative patients	50%
Elderly patients (>70 years) admitted to medical wards	30%–50%

Box 7.1 Impediments in the Recognition of Delirium: Confusion Regarding Terminology

1. Lack of consistency in utilizing diagnostic classification systems
2. The signs and symptoms of delirium can be diverse, and are sometimes mistaken for other psychiatric disorders, such as mood or anxiety disorders.

Box 7.2 Subcategories of Cognitive Disorders According to DSM-IV-TR*[,10]

1. Delirium, dementia, amnesia, and other cognitive disorders
2. Mental disorders caused by a general medical condition (including mood disorder, anxiety disorder, and personality change resulting from a general medical condition)
3. Substance-related disorders

* *Diagnostic and Statistical Manual of Mental Disorders*, 4th ed, text revision.

Box 7.3 Delirium: Morbidity and Mortality

- Delirium is associated with increased morbidity in the terminally ill, causing distress in patients, family members, and staff.[1,3–6,9]
- Delirium can interfere dramatically with the recognition and control of other physical and psychological symptoms such as pain in later stages of illness.[11–13]
- Elderly patients who develop delirium during a hospitalization have been estimated to have a 22% to 76% risk of mortality during that hospitalization.[9]

Box 7.4 The Delirium Experience: Delirium Recall and Delirium-Related Distress[3]

- Fifty-four percent of patients recalled their delirium experience after recovery
- Factors predicting delirium recall included
  - degree of short-term memory impairment,
  - delirium severity, and
  - the presence of perceptual disturbances (the more severe, the less likely the patient was to recall the delirium).
- The most significant factor predicting distress for patients was the presence of delusions. Patients with hypoactive delirium experienced as much distress as patients with hyperactive delirium.
- Predictors of spouse distress included the patients' Karnofsky Performance Status (the lower the Karnofsky score, the worse the spouse distress).
- Predictors of nurse distress included delirium severity and perceptual disturbances.

development of educational interventions to inform patients and caregivers of delirium in palliative care settings.[14]

Delirium is a sign of significant physiological disturbance, usually involving multiple medical etiologies, including infection, organ failure, medication side effects (including opioids), as well as extremely rare paraneoplastic syndromes.[1]

The study of the pathophysiology of delirium is vital to our understanding of the phenomenology, prognosis, treatment, and prevention of delirium. As reflected by its diverse phenomenology, delirium is a dysfunction of multiple regions of the brain, a global cerebral dysfunction. Within the last decade, several hypotheses have been proposed and studied to explain the pathogenesis of delirium. Most hypotheses are complementary rather than competing. It is likely that two or more of these hypotheses act together, leading to syndromes of delirium as opposed to the earlier proposition of a final common pathway. An in-depth review of pathophysiology of delirium is available elsewhere (Boxes 7.5 and 7.6).[8,15]

Clinical Features of Delirium

The clinical features of delirium are quite numerous and include a variety of neuropsychiatric symptoms that are also common to other psychiatric disorders such as depression, dementia, anxiety disorders, and psychosis (Box 7.7).

Box 7.5 Pathophysiology of Delirium: Current Hypotheses[15]

- Oxygen deprivation hypothesis
- Neurotransmitter hypothesis
- Neuronal aging hypothesis
- Neuroendocrine hypothesis
- Inflammatory hypothesis
- Physiological stress hypothesis
- Cellular-signaling hypothesis

Box 7.6 Delirium in the Terminally Ill: Other Considerations[1]

- This is often a pre-terminal event, referred to as "terminal restlessness" or "terminal agitation" in the palliative care literature.
- Reversibility of the process of delirium is often possible in the patient with advanced illness; however, it may not be reversible in the last 24 to 48 hours of life (most likely owing to irreversible processes such as multiple organ failure).[16–18]
- Occasionally delirium may be superimposed on an underlying dementia, as in the case of an elderly patient, an AIDS patient, or a patient with a paraneoplastic syndrome.

Box 7.7 Clinical Features of Delirium[1]

- Prodromal symptoms (restlessness, anxiety, sleep disturbance, and irritability)
- Rapidly fluctuating course
- Attentional disturbances (easily distractible)
- Altered level of alertness
- Increased or decreased psychomotor activity
- Disturbance of sleep-wake cycle
- Affective symptoms (emotional lability, sadness, anger, and euphoria)
- Altered perceptions (misperceptions, illusions, poorly formed delusions, and hallucinations)
- Disorganized thinking and incoherent speech
- Cognitive abnormalities:
  - Disorientation to time, place, or person
  - Memory impairment (cannot register new material)
  - Dysgraphia, constructional apraxia, dysnomic aphasia
- Abnormalities on neurological examination: tremor, asterixis, frontal release signs, myoclonus, and reflex and tone changes
- Electroencephalogram (EEG) abnormalities (usually diffuse slowing)

The essential defining features of delirium, based on DSM-IV-TR[10] criteria, focused on the two essential concepts of disturbances in level of consciousness and attention while continuing to recognize the importance of acute onset and organic etiology (Box 7.8).

Three clinical subtypes of delirium, based on level of alertness and psychomotor behavior, have been described. It is estimated that each subtype comprises approximately one-third of deliria (Boxes 7.9 and 7.10).[19–25]

There is evidence suggesting that specific delirium subtypes may be related to specific etiologies of delirium, may have unique pathophysiologies, and differential responses to treatment.[24–27]

Box 7.8 DSM-IV-TR Criteria for Delirium Caused by a General Medical Condition[10]

- Disturbance of consciousness (reduced clarity or awareness of the environment with reduced ability to focus, sustain, or shift attention)
- Change in cognition (such as memory deficit, disorientation, language disturbance, or perceptual disturbance) that is not better accounted for by a pre-existing, established, or evolving dementia
- The disturbance develops over a short period of time (usually hours to days) and tends to *fluctuate* during the course of the day.
- There is *evidence* from the history, physical examination, or laboratory findings *of a general medical condition* judged to be *etiologically related* to the disturbance.

Box 7.9 Bedside Clinical Examination of Delirium in Palliative Care Settings

Disturbance of Level of Alertness or Awareness

Ask the patient to describe surroundings with eyes closed and ask, "What color is the door?"

Ask the patient, "Are you feeling 100% awake?" and if not, "How awake do you feel?"

Attention Disturbances

Is the patient easily distracted by environmental stimuli or overabsorbed in a task, such as picking at the bed sheet?

Test digit span, starting with 3, 4, then 5 digits forward, followed by 3, 4, then 5 digits backward.

Disorientation

Check for orientation to time, place, and person.

Test the limits of orientation (e.g., year, month, date, day, and time, floor, room number).

Do not assume full orientation because patients know the year and the month.

Cognitive Disturbances

Test registration and immediate recall (use different words for successive evaluations).

Test speech fluency, naming, reading, repetition, writing, comprehension.

Perform clock drawing test.

Perceptual Disturbances (Illusions, Hallucinations)

Ask specifically about hallucinations (e.g., "Are you seeing or hearing strange things?")

Use nursing or family member reports to determine incidents of perceptual disturbances in the course of the day.

Disorganized Thinking

Ask patient an open-ended question (e.g., "Describe your medical condition.")

Listen for rambling, incoherent speech or tangential and circumstantial thought processes.

Delusions

Ask patient, "Are you feeling unsafe here?"

Find out from family or staff whether patient is acting in a paranoid, suspicious, hypervigilant, fearful, or in a hostile fashion.

Psychomotor Disturbances

Observe whether the patient is restless and agitated or slow and hypoactive.

Use observations of family, staff, or both to assess psychomotor activity over previous 24 hours.

Sleep-Wake Cycle Disturbances

Determine from family, staff, or both whether the patient has been "awake most of the night, and asleep most of the day."

(continued)

Box 7.9 (Continued)

Acute Onset, Fluctuating Course
Staff and family are often the best informants. The clinical presentation can be abrupt in onset (e.g., hours to days) and each of the symptoms of delirium can fluctuate over the course of a 24-hour period.
Neurological Signs Consistent with Delirium, such as Asterixis, Frontal Release Signs, and Myoclonus
These findings are supportive of delirium. An electroencephalogram can also be supportive of a delirium diagnosis (diffuse slowing) or can reveal seizure activity.

(Adapted from Breitbart W, Alici Y. Agitation and delirium at the end of life: "We couldn't manage him." *JAMA. 2008*;300:2898–2910.)

Box 7.10 Clinical Subtypes of Delirium[19–25]

1. "*Hyperactive*" (hyperalert, or agitated)—most often characterized by hallucinations, delusions, agitation, and disorientation
2. "*Hypoactive*" (hypoalert, or lethargic)—most often characterized by confusion and sedation; less commonly accompanied by hallucinations, delusions, or illusions*
3. *"Mixed"* (alternating features of hyperactive and hypoactive delirium)

* A recent study by Boettger and Breitbart has shown a prevalence rate of 50.9% of perceptual disturbances and 43.4% of delusions in patients with hypoactive delirium, both of which correlated with presence of moderate to severe disturbance of consciousness and attentional impairment.[23] This further signifies the importance of the diligent management of delirium in patients with all subtypes of delirium to reduce distress and prevent long-term adverse outcomes of delirium.

Many of the clinical features and symptoms of delirium can be also be associated with other psychiatric disorders such as depression, mania, psychosis, and dementia. Delirium, particularly the "hypoactive" subtype, is often initially misdiagnosed as depression, whereas a manic episode may share some features of a "hyperactive" or "mixed" subtype of delirium (Boxes 7.11 and 7.12).

The most common differential diagnostic issue is whether the patient has delirium, or dementia, or a delirium superimposed on a pre-existing dementia. Occasionally one will encounter delirium superimposed on an underlying dementia such as in the case of an elderly patient, an AIDS patient, or a patient with a paraneoplastic syndrome (Box 7.13).[28,29]

Assessment of Delirium

A number of scales or instruments have been developed that can aid the clinician in rapidly screening for cognitive impairment disorders (dementia or delirium), or in establishing a diagnosis of delirium (Box 7.14).

Box 7.11 Guidelines for Distinguishing Delirium from Depression and/or Mania in the Context of Advanced Disease[1,28]

1. Evaluate the onset and temporal sequencing of depressive and cognitive symptoms. Delirium has an abrupt temporal onset.
2. Evaluate the degree of cognitive impairment. The cognitive deficit is much more severe and pervasive in delirium than in depression or mania.
3. Determine whether or not a disturbance in alertness is present. Such a disturbance is not usually a feature of depression or mania.
4. The identification of a presumed medical etiology for delirium is helpful in differentiating these disorders.
5. Paranoid delusions are often present in delirium. Thoughts of guilt, worthlessness, and hopelessness are common in depression. However, frank delusions are rare except in severe depression or mania with psychotic features.
6. Neurological examination is usually normal in patients with mood disorders. In delirium it is not uncommon to find asterixis, positive frontal release signs, and myoclonus.
7. Past history of mood episodes are usually present in patients with a primary mood disorder unlike in patients with delirium.

Box 7.12 Guidelines for Distinguishing Delirium from Psychotic Disorders[1,28]

1. In delirium, psychotic symptoms occur in the context of a disturbance in level of alertness, consciousness, or arousal, as well as memory impairment and disorientation. This is not the case in other psychotic disorders.
2. Delusions in delirium tend to be poorly organized and of abrupt onset.
3. In delirium, hallucinations are predominantly visual or tactile, rather than auditory, as is typical of schizophrenia.
4. The development of these psychotic symptoms in the context of advanced medical illness makes delirium a more likely diagnosis.

Box 7.13 Guidelines for Distinguishing Delirium and Dementia[28,29]

1. The patient with dementia is alert and does not have the disturbance of level of alertness, consciousness, or arousal that is characteristic of delirium.
2. The temporal onset of symptoms in dementia is more subacute and chronically progressive.
3. It is the abrupt onset, fluctuating course, and disturbance in the level of alertness and psychomotor activity that differentiate delirium from dementia.
4. The patient with delirium has more severe sleep-wake cycle disturbance.
5. The most prominent cognitive deficits in dementia include difficulties with short- and long-term memory, impaired judgment, and abstract thinking, as well as disturbed higher cortical functions (e.g., aphasia and apraxia).
6. Delirium, in contrast with dementia, is conceptualized as a reversible process.

Box 7.14 Methods for Assessing Delirium in Patients with Advanced Illness[28,30–40]

Diagnostic Classification Systems
- DSM-IV-TR
- ICD-9, ICD-10
- Research Diagnostic Criteria (RDC)

Diagnostic Interviews/Instruments
- Delirium Symptom Interview (DSI)
- Confusion Assessment Method (CAM)

Confusion Assessment Method-ICU
Cornell Assessment of Pediatric Delirium Assessment (CAP-D)
Intensive Care Delirium Screening Checklist (ICDSC)
NEECHAM Scale
Delirium Detection Score

Delirium Rating Scales
- Delirium Rating Scale (DRS)
- Delirium Rating Scale—Revised—98 (DRS-R-98)
- Confusion Rating Scale (CRS)
- Saskatoon Delirium Checklist (SDC)
- Memorial Delirium Assessment Scale (MDAS)
- Abbreviated Cognitive Test for Delirium (CTD)

Cognitive Impairment Screening Instruments
- Mini-Mental State Exam (MMSE)
- Short Portable Mental Status Questionnaire (SPMSQ)
- Cognitive Capacity Screening Examination (CCSE)
- Blessed Orientation Memory Concentration Test (BOMC)

Montreal Cognitive Assessment Test

Many of these scales have been described and their relative strengths and weaknesses reviewed elsewhere (Box 7.15).[28,20,36,37]

The standard approach to the management of delirium in the medically ill, and even in those with advanced disease, includes a search for underlying causes, correction of those factors, and management of the symptoms of delirium (Figure 7.1).

In the terminally ill patient who develops delirium in the last days of life ("terminal delirium"), the management of delirium is unique, presenting a number of dilemmas. The desired clinical outcome may be significantly altered by the dying process.

When confronted with a delirium in the terminally ill or dying patient, a differential diagnosis should always be formulated as to the likely etiology(ies) (Boxes 7.16 and 7.18).[1]

Hypoxic encephalopathy, hepatic and other organ failure, and disseminated intravascular anticoagulation are less likely to be reversed in terminal delirium (Box 7.18).[17,18]

Box 7.15 Memorial Delirium Assessment Scale[31]

1. Reduced level of consciousness (awareness)
2. Disorientation
3. Short-term memory impairment
4. Impaired digit span
5. Reduced ability to maintain and shift attention
6. Disorganized thinking
7. Perceptual disturbance
8. Delusions
9. Decreased or increased psychomotor
10. Sleep-wake cycle disturbance (disorder of arousal)

* Lawlor et al. found that a cutoff score of 10 yielded the highest sensitivity and specificity for diagnosing delirium in the palliative care population (Lawlor P, Nekolaichuck C, Gagnon B, et al. Clinical utility, factor analysis and further validation of the Memorial Delirium Assessment Scale (MDAS). *Cancer* 2000;88:2859–2867.)

Management of Delirium in Terminally Ill Patients

Clinical experience in managing delirium in dying patients suggests that the short-term, low-dose use of antipsychotics in the management of agitation, paranoia, hallucinations, and altered level of alertness is safe, effective, and often quite appropriate. Only 0.5% to 2% of hospitalized cancer patients receive haloperidol for the management of the symptoms of delirium.[41,42]

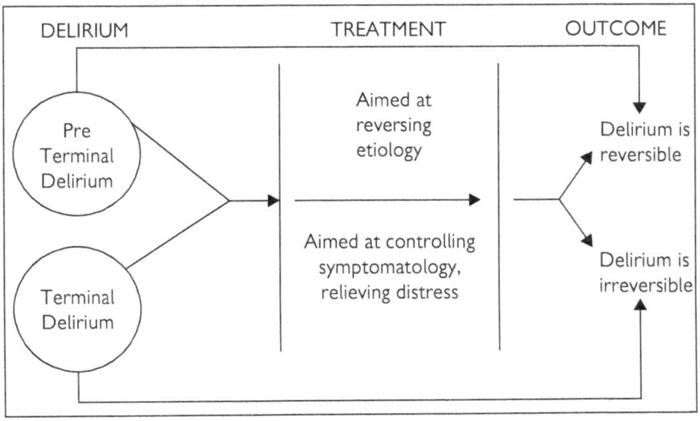

Figure 7.1 Overview of Management of Delirium in Pre-Terminal and Terminally Ill Patients. Adapted from Breitbart W, Lawlor PG, Friedlander M. Delirium in the terminally ill. In: Chochinov HM, Breitbart W, eds. *Handbook of Psychiatry in Palliative Medicine*. New York: Oxford University Press; 2012:81–100.

Box 7.16 Assessment of Delirium Etiology: Guidelines and Considerations[1,2]

1. Undertake diagnostic studies only when a clinically suspected etiology can be identified easily (with minimal use of invasive procedures) and treated effectively (with simple interventions that carry minimal burden or risk of causing further distress).
2. Diagnostic workup in pursuit of an etiology for delirium may be limited by either practical constraints such as the setting (home, hospice) or the focus on patient comfort. Uncomfortable or painful diagnostic procedures should be avoided.
3. Most often, the etiology of terminal delirium is multifactorial, and may not be determined (see Box 7.17).
4. When a distinct cause is found for delirium *in the terminally ill*, it is often irreversible or difficult to treat. In patients with *earlier stages of advanced cancer*, however, a thorough diagnostic assessment can be potentially useful. When such diagnostic information is available, specific therapy may be able to reverse delirium.
5. The diagnostic workup should include an assessment of potentially reversible causes of delirium:
   a. physical exam to assess for evidence of sepsis, dehydration, or major organ failure
   b. review of medications that may potentially contribute to delirium
   c. screen of laboratory parameters to assess the possibility of metabolic abnormalities, hypoxemia, or disseminated intravascular coagulation
   d. imaging studies of the brain and assessment of cerebrospinal fluid may be appropriate in some instances

The readers should refer to the 2012 review by Breitbart and Alici[2] for further information on evidence-based treatment options of delirium in palliative care settings.

The use of antipsychotics and other pharmacological agents in the management of delirium in the dying patient is a standard practice. However, some have argued that pharmacological interventions with antipsychotics or benzodiazepines are inappropriate under certain conditions in the dying patient. Some clinicians believe that certain hallucinations and delusions, particularly those involving dead relatives communicating with dying patients and/or welcoming the dying patient to heaven, are important elements in the transition from life to death. Clearly, there are many patients who experience hallucinations and delusions during delirium that are pleasant or comforting. Some clinicians therefore question the appropriateness of intervening pharmacologically in such instances.

A responsible strategy for utilizing antipsychotics in the management of the symptoms of delirium (e.g., hallucinations that hold religious or spiritual meaning for patients and families) involves two steps: (1) an acknowledgment of

Box 7.17 Potential Etiologies of Delirium[1,2]

Direct Central Nervous System (CNS) Causes
- Primary brain tumor
- Metastatic spread to CNS
- Seizures including non-epileptiform status epilepticus

Indirect Causes
- Metabolic encephalopathy caused by organ failure
- Electrolyte imbalance
- Treatment side effects from:
  - chemotherapeutic agents*
  - narcotic analgesics
  - corticosteroids†
  - radiation therapy
- exogenous cytokines-interferon, interleukin
  - anticholinergics
  - antiemetics
  - antivirals

Other medications and therapeutic modalities
- Infection
- Hematologic abnormalities
- Nutritional deficiencies
- Paraneoplastic syndromes: limbic encephalitis

*Except for ifosfamide and intrathecal methotrexate, most patients receiving these agents will not develop prominent CNS effects.
†The spectrum of mental disturbances related to steroids includes minor mood lability, affective disorders (mania or depression), cognitive impairment (reversible dementia), and delirium (steroid psychosis).

Box 7.18 Commonly Reversible Causes of Delirium[1,17,18]

- Glucocorticosteroids
- Dehydration
- Hypercalcemia
- Psychoactive/opioid medications

respect for a patient/family's beliefs; and (2) an explanation of the unstable and medical nature of delirium. Comforting hallucinations can very rapidly change into frightening and distressing hallucinations. Obtaining permission from a patient or family to utilize antipsychotics under conditions in which the symptoms of delirium become distressing is often possible and ideal (Table 7.2; Boxes 7.19–7.21).

There have not been any trials testing the efficacy and safety of newer antipsychotics (e.g., iloperidone, paliperidone, asenapine) in the treatment of delirium in palliative care settings to the best of our knowledge.

Haloperidol is often the drug of choice in the treatment of delirium in patients with advanced disease (Boxes 7.22 and 7.23).[2]

Box 7.19 Common Misconceptions about Treatment of Delirium in the Terminally Ill

- Patients so close to death should not be treated aggressively.
- Delirium is a natural part of the dying process that should not be altered.
- Parenteral antipsychotics or sedatives may hasten death through hypotension or respiratory depression.
- Pessimism about the possible results of antipsychotic treatment for delirium
- Since the underlying pathophysiological process often continues unabated (e.g., hepatic or renal failure), no improvement can be expected in the symptoms of delirium.
- Antipsychotics may worsen delirium by making the patient more confused or sedated.

Box 7.20 Guidelines for the Treatment of Delirium

1. Delirium should be managed on a case-by-case basis.
2. Symptomatic treatment with antipsychotics or sedative medications is often necessary for the delirious patient with advanced illness.
3. A more cautious approach may be appropriate for patients with a lethargic or somnolent presentation of delirium, or those who are having frankly pleasant or comforting hallucinations. It should be noted, however, that a lethargic or "hypoactive" delirium may very quickly and unexpectedly elevate to an agitated or "hyperactive" delirium that can threaten the serenity and safety of the patient, family, and staff.
4. The use of psychostimulants in the treatment of the hypoactive subtype of delirium in terminally ill patients has been considered. In the absence of randomized controlled trials, psychostimulants cannot be recommended routinely in the treatment of patients with cancer with delirium. However, the use of psychostimulants alone or in combination of antipsychotics should be considered in terminally ill delirium patients with hypoactive delirium who are in significant distress.[43–45]
5. The clinician must consult with the family (and the patient, when lucid) to elicit their concerns and wishes for care during the dying process. The clinician should describe the optimal achievable goals of therapy as they currently exist.
6. If sedation becomes necessary, family members should be informed that the goal of sedation is to provide comfort and symptom control, and not to hasten death. They should also be advised that sedation may result in a premature sense of loss.
7. Ultimately, the clinician must always keep in mind the goals of care and communicate these goals to the staff, patients, and family members. The clinician must consider each of the issues outlined here while preserving and respecting the dignity and values of that individual and family.

Box 7.21 Statements That May Be Helpful to Psycho-oncologists in Guiding Patients and Families through the Course and Treatment of Delirium in Palliative Care Settings

"Delirium develops in very common among patients during the last weeks of life."

"Delirium presents with changes in behavior and thinking, but it is really a sign that multiple medical problems related to the underlying disease are interfering with the brain working normally."

"Delirium is medical in nature; it does not mean that your loved one has now suddenly developed a new psychiatric illness or is having a 'nervous breakdown.'"

"Delirium can be very distressing for patients, families, and staff."

"Delirium can cause agitation or it can cause sedation and sleepiness, and it can be mistaken for depression."

"Delirium can interfere with assessment of symptoms like pain."

"Delirium can be effectively managed, resulting in less distress and better symptom control."

"When you lose the ability to communicate with your loved one because of delirium, it is a terrible loss. It's as if you've lost the essence of who he or she is, and your own grieving process may begin. That's normal and it helps to anticipate that this might occur."

"The goal of treating the symptoms of delirium is to have the patient awake, alert, coherent, and communicating meaningfully with the family and staff, if possible."

"Using sedation to control symptoms at this stage of illness does not shorten survival, it merely provides better comfort."

"We may be running out of time to discuss important treatment preferences together, that is, while your loved one is still able to participate, even minimally, in decision making."

"With the development of delirium at this stage of illness, it may be a good idea to bring to the hospital any family members who are far away and would want to be here if things took a turn for the worse."

"Delirium, in patients with far advanced disease, unfortunately may be a predictor of death in the coming days to weeks."

(Adapted from Breitbart W, Alici Y: Agitation and delirium at the end of life: "We couldn't manage him." *JAMA*. 2008;300:2898–2910.)

Table 7.2 Antipsychotic Medications Used in the Treatment of Delirium

Medication	Dose Range	Routes of Administration	Side Effects	Comments
Typical Antipsychotics				
Haloperidol†	0.5–2 mg every 2–12 h	PO, IV, IM, SC	Extrapyramidal adverse effects can occur at higher doses. Monitor QT interval on EKG.	Remains the gold standard therapy for delirium. May add lorazepam (0.5–1 mg every 2–4 hours) for agitated patients. Double-blind controlled trials support efficacy in treatment of delirium. A pilot placebo-controlled trial suggests lack of efficacy when compared with placebo.
Chlorpromazine†	12.5–50 mg every 4–6 h	PO, IV, IM, SC, PR	More sedating and anticholinergic compared with haloperidol. Monitor blood pressure for hypotension. More suitable for use in ICU settings for closer blood pressure monitoring.	May be preferred in agitated patients due to its sedative effect. Double-blind controlled trials support efficacy in treatment of delirium. No placebo-controlled trials.
Atypical Antipsychotics				
Olanzapine†	2.5–5 mg every 12–24 h	PO*, IM	Sedation is the main dose-limiting adverse effect in short-term use.	Older age, pre-existing dementia, and hypoactive subtype of delirium have been associated with poor response. Double-blind comparison trials with haloperidol and risperidone support efficacy in the treatment of delirium. A pilot placebo-controlled prevention trial suggested worsening in delirium severity. A placebo-controlled study is supportive of efficacy in reducing delirium severity and duration.
Risperidone†	0.25–1 mg every 12–24 h	PO*	Extrapyramidal adverse effects can occur with doses >6 mg/day. Orthostatic hypotension.	Double-blind comparison trials support efficacy in the treatment of delirium. No placebo control trials.

Quetiapine†	12.5–100 mg every 12–24 h	PO	Sedation, orthostatic hypotension.	Sedating effects may be helpful in patients with sleep-wake cycle disturbance. Pilot placebo-controlled trials suggest efficacy in treatment of delirium. However, studies allowed for concomitant use of haloperidol, which makes the results difficult to interpret.
Ziprasidone	10–40 mg every 12–24 h	PO, IM	Monitor QT interval on EKG.	Placebo-controlled, double-blind trial suggests lack of efficacy in the treatment of delirium.
Aripiprazole‡	5–30 mg every 24 h	PO*, IM	Monitor for akathisia.	Evidence is limited. A prospective open label trial suggests comparable efficacy to haloperidol. There is some evidence to suggest its efficacy in hypoactive subtype of delirium. No placebo-controlled trials.

* Risperidone, olanzapine, and aripiprazole are available in orally disintegrating tablets. There have been no intervention or prevention trials with the use of recently released antipsychotics, including paliperidone, iloperidone, asenapine, or lurasidone in the treatment or prevention of delirium.
† Despite shortcomings of the studies described in the text, there is US Preventive Services Task Force (USPSTF) Level I evidence for the use of haloperidol, risperidone, olanzapine, and quetiapine in the treatment of delirium.
‡ There is USPSTF Level II-2 evidence for the use of aripiprazole in the treatment of delirium.
(Adapted from Breitbart W, Alici Y. Evidence-based treatment of delirium in patients with cancer. *J Clin Oncol* 2012;30:1206–1214.)[1,2,46–59]

Box 7.22 Haloperidol and Other Typical Antipsychotics[2,28]

- In low doses (1–3 mg), haloperidol is usually effective in targeting agitation, paranoia, and fear. Typically 0.5 mg to 1.0 mg (PO, IV, IM, SC) is administered, with repeat doses every 45 to 60 minutes titrated against target symptoms.
- An intravenous route can facilitate rapid onset of medication effects. If intravenous access is unavailable, one can start with intramuscular or subcutaneous administration and switch to the oral route when possible.
- The majority of delirious patients can be managed with oral haloperidol.
- Parenteral doses are approximately twice as potent as oral doses.
- Delivery of haloperidol by the subcutaneous route is utilized by many palliative care practitioners.
- In elderly patients, low doses of antipsychotic medications are usually sufficient in treating delirium. In general, doses need not to exceed 20 mg of haloperidol in a 24-hour period; however, some authors have advocated high doses (up to 250 mg/24 hour of haloperidol, usually IV) in selected cases.[60]
- Parenteral lorazepam is often added to a regimen of haloperidol in order to more rapidly and effectively sedate the agitated delirious patient.[2] The addition of lorazepam may also help minimize extrapyramidal side effects associated with haloperidol. Lorazepam alone, however, is ineffective in the treatment of delirium and in fact, may contribute to worsening delirium and cognitive impairment.[46]
- An alternative strategy is to switch from haloperidol to a more sedating antipsychotic, such as chlorpromazine, which may significantly improve the symptoms of delirium in both the "hypoactive" and "hyperactive" states.[2,46]
- Evidence suggests that the subtypes of delirium may have different treatment responses. A randomized controlled trial of haloperidol and chlorpromazine found that both medications were equally effective in hypoactive and hyperactive subtypes of delirium.[46]

Box 7.23 Atypical or Second-Generation Antipsychotics

- A 2004 Cochrane review on drug therapy for delirium in the terminally ill concluded that haloperidol was the most suitable medication for the treatment of patients with delirium near the end of life, with chlorpromazine being an acceptable alternative.[49]
- A 2007 Cochrane review comparing the efficacy and incidence of adverse effects between haloperidol and atypical antipsychotics concluded that, like haloperidol, selected atypical antipsychotics (risperidone and olanzapine) were effective in managing delirium.[48] Haloperidol doses greater than 4.5 mg/d resulted in increased rates of extrapyramidal symptoms compared with the atypical antipsychotics, but low-dose haloperidol (i.e., 3.5 mg/d) was not shown to result in a greater frequency of extrapyramidal adverse effects.[48,50,51]

(continued)

Box 7.23 (Continued)

- None of the antipsychotics were found to be superior when compared with others in the treatment of delirium symptoms, and there is evidence for efficacy in the improvement of the symptoms of delirium for the following atypical antipsychotics: olanzapine, risperidone, aripiprazole, and quetiapine.[2,48,59]
- Two open-label trials showed different treatment responses to different antipsychotics. In one open-label trial,[26] the hypoactive subtype was associated with poorer treatment response to olanzapine. Another open-label study[27] suggested that the hypoactive subtype of delirium was associated with better response to treatment with aripiprazole.
- To the best of our knowledge there have not been any studies testing the safety and efficacy of parenteral forms of atypical antipsychotics, namely, olanzapine and aripiprazole that have become available in the intramuscular forms within the last few years.

Although antipsychotic drugs such as haloperidol are most effective in diminishing agitation, clearing the sensorium, and improving cognition in the delirious patient, this is not always possible in delirium that complicates the last days of life. Up to 10% to 20% of terminally ill patients experience delirium that can only be controlled by sedation to the point of a significantly decreased level of consciousness.[61–70]

As outlined in detail in a comprehensive review of evidence-based treatment of delirium in cancer patients,[2] the following monitoring guidelines are recommended for patients with delirium treated with antipsychotic medications. Recommendations are based on the Consensus Development Conference on antipsychotic drugs and obesity and diabetes.[71] However, it is important to note that the risks and benefits of carrying out the laboratory testing should be individualized not to burden the patients with unnecessary blood draws or other procedures at the end of life (Boxes 7.24 and 7.25).

In addition to seeking out and potentially correcting underlying causes for delirium, symptomatic and supportive therapies are important (Box 7.26).

Summary[2]

- Current evidence is supportive of short-term use of antipsychotics in the treatment of symptoms of delirium (i.e., agitation, sleep-wake cycle disturbances, delusions, hallucinations) with close monitoring for possible adverse effects, especially in elderly patients with multiple medical comorbidities.
- The longest clinical and research experience and safety/efficacy data available are for haloperidol. Low-dose haloperidol is still considered the gold standard in treatment of delirium. There is growing evidence for the efficacy of atypical antipsychotics in the management of delirium as well. The choice of antipsychotic medication for the treatment of delirium should be based on the clinical presentation of the patient and the adverse effect profile of each

Box 7.24 Monitoring Guidelines for Patients with Delirium on Antipsychotic Medications

ECG: Baseline, and with every dose increase (consider daily monitoring if on high doses [e.g., haloperidol >5–10 mg daily], patients with underlying unstable cardiac disease, patients with electrolyte disturbances, patients on other QT prolonging medications,* medically frail, older patients; patients with unstable cardiac diseases or those on intravenous antipsychotics may require continuous monitoring in consultation with cardiology.)

Fasting lipid profile: Baseline and every 3 months

Fasting blood glucose: Baseline and weekly

Body mass index: Baseline and weekly

Extrapyramidal adverse effects (including Parkinsonism, dystonia, akathisia, neuroleptic malignant syndrome): Baseline, and daily

Blood pressure, pulse: Baseline and at least daily (High-risk patients should be monitored more closely. Continuous monitoring may be required in medically unstable patients. Orthostatic measurements should be considered with antipsychotics with alpha-1 antagonist effects, such as chlorpromazine and risperidone.)

(Adapted from Breitbart W, Alici Y. Evidence-based treatment of delirium in patients with cancer. *J Clin Oncol* 2012;*30:1206–1214.)*

* The risk of QT prolongation is directly correlated with higher antipsychotic doses, with parenteral formulations (e.g., intravenous haloperidol) of antipsychotics, and with certain medications (e.g., ziprasidone, thioridazine).[72–74] In individual patients, an absolute QTc interval of 500 ms or an increase of 60 ms (or > 20%) from baseline is regarded as indicating an increased risk of torsades des pointes.[73] Discontinuation of the antipsychotic and a consultation with a cardiologist should be considered, especially if there is continued need for the use of antipsychotics.

Box 7.25 Sedation as a Goal of Delirium Treatment[61–70]

- The goal of treatment with such agents as midazolam and propofol is quiet sedation only.
- Before undertaking interventions, such as midazolam or propofol infusions, where the best achievable goal is a calm and comfortable but sedated and unresponsive patient, the clinician must review the diagnosis, prognosis, treatment options, and individualized goals of care with the family and the patient if at all possible.
- In studies of the use of palliative sedation for symptom control, delirium was identified as the target symptom in up to 36% of cases.
- Propofol has an advantage over midazolam in that the level of sedation is more easily controlled and recovery is rapid upon decreasing the rate of infusion.
- The ethical concerns of palliative sedation have been reviewed in an article by Lo and Rubenfeld.[66]

Box 7.26 Nonpharmacological Interventions for Delirium

Reviewing medication list to avoid polypharmacy
Controlling pain
Promoting good sleep pattern and sleep hygiene
Monitoring closely for dehydration and fluid-electrolyte disturbances
Monitoring nutrition
Monitoring for sensory deficits, providing visual and hearing aids
Avoiding immobility, encouraging early mobilization (minimizing the use of immobilizing catheters, intravenous lines, and physical restraints)*
Monitoring bowel and bladder function
Reorienting the patient frequently
Placing an orientation board, clock, or familiar objects in patient rooms
Encouraging cognitively stimulating activities

(Adapted from Breitbart W, Alici Y. Evidence-based treatment of delirium in patients with cancer. *J Clin Oncol* 2012;30:1206–1214.)[2,75–77]

* Physical restraints should be avoided both in patients who are at risk for developing delirium and those who have delirium. The use of physical restraints has been identified as an independent risk factor for delirium persistence at the time of hospital discharge.[75] Restraint-free care should be the standard of care for prevention and treatment of delirium among cancer patients.

antipsychotic drug, given that none of the antipsychotics were found to be superior to others in comparison trials.

- It is strongly recommended to implement nonpharmacological interventions in the routine care of patients who are at risk for delirium and of patients with established delirium, based on the evidence from non-oncology settings. There are no known risks associated with the use of nonpharmacological interventions.
- There is no evidence to support the use of cholinesterase inhibitors in treatment or prevention of delirium in palliative care settings. The use of psychostimulants in the treatment of hypoactive subtype of delirium in terminally ill patients has been considered. In the absence of randomized controlled trials psychostimulants cannot currently be recommended in the treatment of patients with cancer with delirium.
- Current evidence is not supportive of the use of antipsychotics for the prevention of delirium in patients with cancer.
- The evidence supporting the use of intravenous dexmedetomidine for the prevention of delirium has been mixed and is limited to patients in intensive care settings only; there is currently no evidence to support its use in palliative care settings as a treatment for delirium.

References

1. Breitbart W, Alici Y. Agitation and delirium at the end of life: "We couldn't manage him." *JAMA*. 2008;300:2898–2910.

2. Breitbart W, Alici Y. Evidence-based treatment of delirium in patients with cancer. *J Clin Oncol.* 2012;30:1206–1214.
3. Breitbart W, Gibson C, Tremblay A. The delirium experience: delirium recall and delirium related distress in hospitalized patients with cancer, their spouses/caregivers, and their nurses. *Psychosomatics* 2002;43:183–194.
4. Morita T, Hirai K, Sakaguchi Y, et al. Family perceived distress from delirium-related symptoms of terminally ill cancer patients. *Psychosomatics* 2004;45:107–113.
5. Bruera E, Bush SH, Willey J, et al. Impact of delirium and recall on the level of distress in patients with advanced cancer and their family caregivers. *Cancer* 2009;115(9):2004–2012.
6. Buss MK, Vanderwerker LC, Inouye SK, Zhang B, Block SD, Prigerson HG. Associations between caregiver-perceived delirium in patients with cancer and generalized anxiety in their caregivers. *J Palliat Med.* 2007;10(5):1083–1092.
7. Fann JR, Roth-Roemer S, Burington BE, et al. Delirium in patients undergoing hematopoietic stem cell transplantation. *Cancer* 2002;95:1971–1981.
8. Maldonado JR. Pathoetiological model of delirium: a comprehensive understanding of the neurobiology of delirium and an evidence-based approach to prevention and treatment. *Crit Care Clin.* 2008;24:789–856.
9. Inouye SK. Delirium in older persons. *N Engl J Med.* 2006;354:1157–1165.
10. American Psychiatric Association. *Diagnostic and Statistical Manual of Mental Disorders*, 4th ed. Washington, DC: American Psychiatric Association Press; 2000.
11. Gagnon B, Lawlor PG, Mancini IL, Pereira JL, Hanson J, Bruera ED. The impact of delirium on the circadian distribution of breakthrough analgesia in advanced cancer patients. *J Pain Symptom Manage.* 2001;22(4):826–833.
12. Coyle N, Breitbart W, Weaver S, Portenoy R. Delirium as a contributing factor to 'Crescendo' pain: three case reports. *J Pain Symptom Manage.* 1994;9:44–47.
13. Morita T, Tei Y, Inouye S. Impaired communication capacity and agitated delirium in the final week of terminally ill cancer patients: prevalence and identification of research focus. *J Pain Symptom Manage.* 2003;26:827–834.
14. Gagnon P, Charbonneau C, Allard P, Soulard C, Dumont S, Fillion L. Delirium in advanced cancer: a psychoeducational intervention for family caregivers. *J Palliat Care.* 2002;18(4):253–261.
15. Steiner LA. Postoperative delirium. Part 1: pathophysiology and risk factors. *Eur J Anaesthesiol.* 2011;28(9):628–636.
16. Leonard M, Raju B, Conroy M, et al. Reversibility of delirium in terminally ill patients and predictors of mortality. *Palliat Med.* 2008;22(7):848–854.
17. Morita T, Tei Y, Tsunoda J, Inoue S, Chihara S. Underlying pathologies and their associations with clinical features in terminal delirium of cancer patients. *J Pain Symptom Manage.* 2001;22(6):997–1006.
18. Lawlor P, Gagnon B, Mancini I, et al. The occurrence, causes and outcomes of delirium in advanced cancer patients: a prospective study. *Arch Intern Med.* 2002;160:786–794.
19. Meagher DJ, O'Hanlon D, O'Mahony E, Casey PR, Trzepacz PT. Relationship between symptoms and motoric subtype of delirium. *J Neuropsychiatry Clin Neurosci.* 2000;12(1):51–56.
20. Stagno D, Gibson C, Breitbart W. The delirium subtypes: a review of prevalence, phenomenology, pathophysiology, and treatment response. *Palliat Support Care.* 2004;2(2):171–179.

21. Fang CK, Chen HW, Liu SI, Lin CJ, Tsai LY, Lai YL. Prevalence, detection and treatment of delirium in terminal cancer inpatients: a prospective survey. *Jpn J Clin Oncol.* 2008;38(1):56–63.

22. Leonard M, Donnelly S, Conroy M, Trzepacz P, Meagher DJ. Phenomenological and neuropsychological profile across motor variants of delirium in a palliative-care unit. *J Neuropsychiatry Clin Neurosci.* 2011;23(2):180–188.

23. Boettger S, Breitbart W. Phenomenology of the subtypes of delirium: Phenomenological differences between hyperactive and hypoactive delirium. *Palliat Support Care* 2011;9:129–135.

24. Spiller JA, Keen JC. Hypoactive delirium: assessing the extent of the problem for inpatient specialist palliative care. *Palliat Med.* 2006;20(1):17–23.

25. Kiely DK, Jones RN, Bergmann MA, Marcantonio ER. Association between psychomotor activity delirium subtypes and mortality among newly admitted post-acute facility patients. *J Gerontol A Biol Sci Med Sci.* 2007;62(2):174–179.

26. Breitbart W, Tremblay A, Gibson C. An open trial of olanzapine for the treatment of delirium in hospitalized cancer patients. *Psychosomatics* 2002;43(3):175–182.

27. Boettger S, Friedlander M, Breitbart W, et al. Aripiprazole and haloperidol in the treatment of delirium. *Aust N Z J Psychiatry* 2011;45:477–482.

28. American Psychiatric Association. Practice guidelines for the treatment of patients with delirium. *Am J Psychiatry.* 1999;156(5 suppl):1–20.

29. Boettger S, Passik S, Breitbart W. Delirium superimposed on dementia versus delirium in the absence of dementia: phenomenological differences. *Palliat Support Care.* 2009;7(4):495–500.

30. Smith MJ, Breitbart WS, Platt MM. A critique of instruments and methods to detect, diagnose, and rate delirium. *J Pain Symptom Manage.* 1994;10(1):35–77.

31. Breitbart W, Rosenfeld B, Roth A. The Memorial Delirium Assessment Scale. *J Pain Symptom Manage.* 1997;13:128–137.

32. Lawlor P, Nekolaichuck C, Gagnon B, et al. Clinical utility, factor analysis and further validation of the Memorial Delirium Assessment Scale (MDAS). *Cancer* 2000;88:2859–2867.

33. Trzepacz PT, Mittal D, Torres R, Kanary K, Norton J, Jimerson N. Validation of the Delirium Rating Scale-revised-98: comparison with the delirium rating scale and the cognitive test for delirium. *J Neuropsychiatry Clin Neurosci.* 2001;13(2):229–242.

34. Inouye B, Vandyck C, Alessi C. Clarifying confusion: the confusion assessment method, a new method for the detection of delirium. *Ann Intern Med.* 1990;113:941–948.

35. Ryan K, Leonard M, Guerin S, et al. Validation of the confusion assessment method in the palliative care setting. *Palliat Med.* 2009;23:40–55.

36. Wong CL, Holroyd-Leduc J, Simel DL, Straus SE. Does this patient have delirium? Value of bedside instruments. *JAMA.* 2010;304(7):779–786.

37. Devlin JW, Fong JJ, Fraser GL, Riker RR. Delirium assessment in the critically ill. *Int Care Med.* 2007;33:929–940.

38. Csokasy J. Assessment of acute confusion: use of the NEECHAM Confusion Scale. *Appl Nurs Res.* 1999;12:51–55.

39. Immers HE, Schuurmans MJ, van de Bijl JJ. Recognition of delirium in ICU patients: a diagnostic study of the NEECHAM confusion scale in ICU patients. *BMC Nurs.* 2005;4:7.

40. Otter H, Martin J, Basell K, von Heymann C, Hein OV, Bollert P, et al. Validity and reliability of the DDS for severity of delirium in the ICU. *Neurocrit Care* 2005;2:150–158.

41. Derogatis L, Feldstein M, Morrow G. A survey of psychotropic drug prescriptions in an oncology population. *Cancer* 1979;44:1919–1929.

42. Stiefel F, Kornblith A, Holland J. Changes in the prescription patterns of psychotropic drugs for cancer patients during a 10 year period. *Cancer* 1990;65:1048–1053.

43. Gagnon B, Low G, Schreier G. Methylphenidate hydrochloride improves cognitive function in patients with advanced cancer and hypoactive delirium: a prospective clinical study. *J Psychiatry Neurosci.* 2005;30:100–107.

44. Keen JC, Brown D. Psychostimulants and delirium in patients receiving palliative care. *Palliat Support Care* 2004;2:199–202.

45. Morita T, Otani H, Tsunoda J, et al. Successful palliation of hypoactive delirium due to multi-organ failure by oral methylphenidate. *Support Care Cancer* 2000;8:134–137.

46. Breitbart W, Marotta R, Platt M. A double-blind comparison trial of haloperidol, chlorpromazine, and lorazepam in the treatment of delirium in hospitalized AIDS patients. *Am J Psychiatry* 1996;153:231–237.

47. Boettger S, Breitbart W. Atypical antipsychotics in the management of delirium: a review of the empirical literature. *Palliat Support Care* 2005;3:227–237.

48. Lonergan E, Britton AM, Luxenberg J, et al. Antipsychotics for delirium. *Cochrane Database Syst Rev* 2007;2:CD005594.

49. Jackson KC, Lipman AG. Drug therapy for delirium in terminally ill patients. *Cochrane Database Syst Rev* 2004;2:CD004770.

50. Han CS, Kim YK. A double-blind trial of risperidone and haloperidol for the treatment of delirium. *Psychosomatics* 2004;45:297–301.

51. Hu H, Deng W, Yang H. A prospective random control study: comparison of olanzapine and haloperidol in senile delirium. *Chongqing Med J* 2004;8:1234–1237.

52. Grover S, Kumar V, Chakrabarti S. Comparative efficacy study of haloperidol, olanzapine and risperidone in delirium. *J Psychosom Res.* 2011;71:277–281.

53. Girard TD, Pandharipande PP, Carson SS, et al. Feasibility, efficacy, and safety of antipsychotics for intensive care unit delirium: the MIND randomized, placebo-controlled trial. *Crit Care Med.* 2010;38:428–437.

54. Devlin JW, Roberts RJ, Fong JJ, et al. Efficacy and safety of quetiapine in critically ill patients with delirium: a prospective, multicenter, randomized, double-blind, placebo-controlled pilot study. *Crit Care Med.* 2010;38:419–427.

55. Tahir TA, Eeles E, Karapareddy V, et al. A randomized controlled trial of quetiapine versus placebo in the treatment of delirium. *J Psychosom Res.* 2010;69:485–490.

56. Elsayem A, Bush SH, Munsell MF, et al. Subcutaneous olanzapine for hyperactive or mixed delirium in patients with advanced cancer: a preliminary study. *J Pain Symptom Manage.* 2010;40:774–782.

57. Kim SW, Yoo JA, Lee SY, et al. Risperidone versus olanzapine for the treatment of delirium. *Hum Psychopharmacol.* 2010;25:298–302.

58. Kim KY, Bader GM, Kotlyar V, et al. Treatment of delirium in older adults with quetiapine. *J Geriatr Psychiatry Neurol.* 2003;16:29–31.

59. Flaherty JH. The evaluation and management of delirium among older persons. *Med Clin North Am.* 2011;95:555–577.

60. Fernandez F, Holmes V, Adams F, Kavanaugh J. Treatment of severe refractory agitation with a Haldol drip. *J Clin Psychiatry* 1988;49:239–241.

61. Ventafridda V, Ripamonti C, DeConno F, Tamburini M, Cassileth BR. Symptom prevalence and control during cancer patients' last days of life. *J Palliat Care.* 1990;6(3):7–11.

62. Fainsinger RL, Waller A, Bercovici M, et al. A multicentre international study of sedation for uncontrolled symptoms in terminally ill patients. *Palliat Med.* 2000;14(4):257–265.

63. Rietjens JA, van Zuylen L, van Veluw H, van der Wijk L, van der Heide A, van der Rijt CC. Palliative sedation in a specialized unit for acute palliative care in a cancer hospital: comparing patients dying with and without palliative sedation. *J Pain Symptom Manage.* 2008;36(3):228–234.

64. Connor SR, Pyenson B, Fitch K, Spence C, Iwasaki K. Comparing hospice and nonhospice patient survival among patients who die within a three-year window. *J Pain Symptom Manage.* 2007;33(3):238–246.

65. Mercadante S, DeConno F, Ripamonti C. Propofol in terminal care. *J Pain Symptom Manage.* 1995;10(8):639–642.

66. Lo B, Rubenfeld G. Palliative sedation in dying patients: "we turn to it when everything else hasn't worked." *JAMA.* 2005;294(14):1810–1816.

67. Sykes N, Thorns A. Sedative use in the last week of life and the implications for end-of-life decision making. *Arch Intern Med.* 2003;163(3):341–344.

68. Morita T, Chinone Y, Ikenaga M, et al. Efficacy and safety of palliative sedation therapy: a multicenter, prospective, observational study conducted on specialized palliative care units in Japan. *J Pain Symptom Manage.* 2005;30(4):320–328.

69. Bercovitch M, Adunsky A. Patterns of high-dose morphine use in a home-care hospice service: should we be afraid of it? *Cancer.* 2004;101(6):1473–1477.

70. Vitetta L, Kenner D, Sali A. Sedation and analgesia-prescribing patterns in terminally ill patients at the end of life. *Am J Hosp Palliat Care.* 2005;22(6):465–473.

71. American Diabetes Association, American Psychiatric Association, American Association of Clinical Endocrinologists, et al. Consensus development conference on antipsychotic drugs and obesity and diabetes. *Diabetes Care* 2004;27:596–601.

72. Harrigan EP, Miceli JJ, Anziano R, et al. A randomized evaluation of the effects of six antipsychotic agents on QTc, in the absence and presence of metabolic inhibition. *J Clin Psychopharmacol.* 2004;24:62–69.

73. Haddad PM, Anderson IM. Antipsychotic-related QTc prolongation, torsade de pointes and sudden death. *Drugs* 2002;62:1649–1671.

74. US Food and Drug Administration. Information for healthcare professionals: Haloperidol (marketed as Haldol, Haldol Decanoate and Haldol Lactate). http:// www.fda.gov/Drugs/DrugSafety/PostmarketDrug SafetyInformationforPatientsandProviders/Drug SafetyInformationforHeathcare Professionals/ucm 085203.htm

75. Inouye SK, Zhang Y, Jones RN, Kiely DK, Yang F, Marcantonio ER, et al. Risk factors for delirium at discharge: development and validation of a predictive model. *Arch Intern Med.* 2007;167:1406–1413.

76. National Institute for Health and Clinical Excellence. Delirium: diagnosis, prevention and management (clinical guideline 103). www.nice.org.uk/nicemedia/live/13060/49909/49909.pdf Accessed August 14, 2012.

77. Gagnon P, Allard P, Gagnon B, Mérette C, Tardif F. Delirium prevention in terminal cancer: assessment of a multicomponent intervention. *Psychooncology* 2010;21(2):187–194.

78. Breitbart W, Lawlor PG, Friedlander M. Delirium in the terminally ill. In: Chochinov HM, Breitbart W, eds. *Handbook of Psychiatry in Palliative Medicine*. New York: Oxford University Press; 2012:81–100.

Part III

Psychosocial Issues in the Palliative Care Setting

Chapter 8

Management of Fatigue in Palliative Care Settings

Fatigue is defined as a subjective feeling of tiredness, generalized weakness, or lack of energy.[1] There is no universally accepted definition of fatigue. Cancer-related fatigue is defined by the National Comprehensive Cancer Network[2] as a distressing, persistent, subjective sense of physical, emotional, and/or cognitive tiredness or exhaustion related to cancer and/or cancer treatment that is not proportional to recent activity and interferes with usual functioning. Fatigue is highly prevalent in palliative care settings. Studies suggest that as many as 60% to 90% of advanced cancer patients complain of fatigue. Fatigue is frequently under-recognized and undertreated in the terminally ill. Further information on assessment and management of fatigue in palliative care settings can be found elsewhere (Box 8.1).[2]

Like pain, fatigue is highly prevalent in palliative care settings. Pain and fatigue frequently coexist and impact patients' quality of life. Fatigue is under-recognized and undertreated at the end of life.[3] As the subjective reporting is of utmost importance in assessment of fatigue, good physician-patient communication is essential to timely recognition and treatment of fatigue among terminally ill patients (Box 8.2).

It is strongly recommended that all health care providers should routinely screen for the presence of fatigue from the point of diagnosis onward. All patients should be screened for fatigue as clinically indicated and at least annually. Screening should be performed and documented using a quantitative or semiquantitative assessment (Boxes 8.3 and 8.4).[2–5]

Box 8.1 Prevalence of Selected Symptoms in Cancer Patients[3]

Physical and psychological symptoms range from 8 to 13 per patients on average and increase with advanced disease.

Pain: 15%–90%
Fatigue: 40%–80%
Anorexia: 40%–55%
Insomnia: 53%
Worrying: 73%
Feeling sad: 68%
Irritability: 47%

Box 8.2 Prevalence* of Cancer-Related Fatigue (CRF) among Patients with Cancer[2–5]

During treatment and in late stages of disease: 60% to 96%
During chemotherapy: 80% to 96%
Among cancer survivors: 30% to 40%

* The use of stricter International Classification of Diseases (ICD) criteria reduces the prevalence of clinically significant CRF by half.

Box 8.3 Selected Instruments Used in Screening and Measurement of Fatigue[6]

Brief Screening Tools

- Visual Analog Scales (VAS)
- Multisymptom screening scales: Edmonton Symptom Assessment Scale[7] Memorial Symptom Assessment Scale[4]

Unidimensional Scales (measure the physical impact of fatigue)

- Functional Assessment of Cancer Therapy-Fatigue (FACT-F)[8]
- Brief Fatigue Inventory (BFI)[9]
- European Organization for Research and Treatment of Cancer Quality of Life Questionnaire (EORTC QLQ C30)[10]
- Profile of Mood States Fatigue (POMSF)[11]

Multidimensional Scales (measure the cognitive, affective, and physical impact of fatigue)

- Fatigue Symptom Inventory[12]
- Revised Piper Fatigue Scale[13]
- Multidimensional Fatigue Inventory[14]
- Schwartz Cancer Fatigue Scale[15]

Assessment of fatigue in palliative care settings should start with a focused fatigue history and physical examination.[2] Fatigue history should include:

- Onset, pattern, duration
- Change over time
- Associated or alleviating factors

Clinicians should evaluate disease status to determine any cancer (i.e., progression of disease, recurrence) or cancer treatment–related changes contributing to fatigue.

As detailed in Box 8.5, clinicians should assess for contributing factors with close attention to those that are treatable (Box 8.6).

Depression should be ruled out in all patients presenting with fatigue (Box 8.7).

Box 8.4 ICD-10 Criteria for Cancer-Related Fatigue[16]

Diagnosis is made if six or more of the following symptoms are present daily or nearly daily during same two weeks in the past month and at least one of the symptoms is significant fatigue:

- Fatigue (diminished energy, increased need to rest disproportionate to change in activity)
- Generalized weakness, limb heaviness
- Diminished concentration
- Decreased motivation, interest in activities
- Insomnia, hypersomnia
- Sleep unrefreshing, unrestorative
- Struggle to overcome activity
- Emotional reactivity to feeling fatigued (sadness, frustration, irritability)
- Difficulty with daily tasks because of fatigue
- Short-term memory problems
- Postexertional malaise lasting several hours

Symptoms cause clinically significant distress or impairment in social, occupational, or other important areas of functioning

Evidence from history, physical examination, or laboratory findings that symptoms are consequence of cancer or cancer therapy

Symptoms are not primarily consequences of comorbid psychiatric disorders such as major depression, somatization or somatoform disorder, or delirium

Box 8.5 Common Contributing Factors of Fatigue in Patients with Advanced Illness[1,2,5,18]

- Pre-existing conditions (congestive heart failure, chronic obstructive pulmonary disease)
- Direct effects of cancer ("tumor burden")
- Cancer treatment effects (surgery, radiation, chemotherapy)
- Emotional distress (anxiety, depression, stress)
- Immobility/deconditioning
- Symptoms of advanced illness (pain, nausea, etc.)
- Disruptions in sleep-wake cycle
- Conditions related to cancer or its treatment (anemia, dehydration, malnutrition, infection, endocrine problems: low testosterone, low thyroid)
- Medications (analgesics, psychotropics, beta-blockers, antiemetics)
- Alcohol and substance abuse
- Nutritional issues

Box 8.6 Strategies for Managing Fatigue[1,2,17–24]

Patient and family/caregiver education: Communication about the availability, effectiveness, and safety of interventions for fatigue must be fostered between patients and health care providers:

- Discussion of the prevalence of fatigue in palliative care settings
- Expected fatigue patterns
- Self-monitoring of fatigue levels
- Importance of reporting fatigue to health care professionals
- Communication about the availability, effectiveness, and safety of interventions for fatigue must be fostered between patients and health care providers.
- An ongoing supportive relationship permits the patient to express fears and concerns about the meaning of continued weakness. The clinician is also able to address distorted ideas that the patient may have about the prognostic significance of fatigue.

Treat underlying physiological and psychological contributing factors of fatigue:

- Treat anemia.
- Treat metabolic abnormalities, nutritional and vitamin deficiencies, hypothyroidism, and hypogonadism.
- Treat anxiety and depression.
- Treat sleep disturbances.
- Eliminate nonessential centrally acting drugs.

Treat fatigue directly:

- Increase or restore energy.
- Conserve energy.
- Improve fatigue and functioning with nonpharmacological and pharmacological interventions.

Manage consequences of fatigue:

- Minimize the negative impact on quality of life. (Maintain important activities even if assistance is needed. Facilitate adjustment to limitations caused by fatigue. Restructure goals and expectations. Assist patients in sustaining sense of meaning.)

When depression and fatigue are comorbid, treatment of the underlying depression takes precedence. Selective serotonin reuptake inhibitors (SSRIs) are better tolerated in comparison with tricyclic antidepressants and monoamine oxidase inhibitors.[2,17,24] Bupropion is more activating, and may be preferred in depressed patients with fatigue (Boxes 8.8–8.11).[2,24]

There is evidence from meta-analytic reviews that psychostimulants provide significant improvement in fatigue at clinically meaningful levels.[2,18–20,23,24] Evidence suggests that psychostimulants (e.g., methylphenidate) and other wakefulness agents (e.g., modafinil) can be effectively used to manage fatigue in

Box 8.7 Differentiating Fatigue and Depression in Palliative Care Settings[2,17]

Several signs and symptoms are common to depression and fatigue such as fatigue, decreased energy, increased need to rest, anhedonia, decreased motivation, sadness, frustration, irritability, insomnia, hypersomnia, concentration and attention deficits, and perceived short-term memory problems.

Fatigue is much more common than depression (60%–90% vs. 20%–25%)

Depressive symptoms due to fatigue are often less severe and are attributed to consequences of fatigue by patients

Depression is more likely in the presence of

- Hopelessness, worthlessness, guilt
- Suicidal ideation, desire for death
- History or family history of depression

Box 8.8 Nonpharmacological Management of Fatigue in Palliative Care Settings[22,25–30]

Physical activity[21,25,27]

Energy conservation and restoration

- Set priorities.
- Pace energy-consuming activities.
- Obtain appropriate rest.
- Delegate, and use labor-saving devices.
- Engage in attention-restoring activities.
- Participate in enjoyable activities.

Sleep restoration

Psychotherapies

- Cognitive behavioral therapy
- Psychoeducation
- Supportive counseling

Meditation, relaxation, yoga, mindfulness based stress reduction, massage, tai chi, music therapy, Reiki, medical qigong

Acupuncture

Nutritional counseling

patients with advanced disease or those on active treatment. However, there is very limited evidence of their effectiveness in reducing fatigue in patients following active treatment who are currently disease free. Further studies are required to confirm these recommendations, as clinical trials have shown mixed results (Table 8.1).

The subgroup analyses of the fatigue intervention trials have shown that patients with advanced disease or more severe fatigue did significantly better

Box 8.9 Pharmacological Interventions for Management of Fatigue in Palliative Care Settings*[2,19,20,23,24]

Psychostimulants
Corticosteroids
Anticytokine agents (thalidomide, pentoxifylline, cox-2 inhibitors)
Other agents (donepezil, carnitine, megestrol acetate, amantadine, anabolic steroids, antidepressants, sleep aids)
Supplements (ginseng, Vitamin D, others)

* Based on the current literature none of the preceding medications could be recommended for use in terminally ill fatigue patients except for psychostimulants.

Box 8.10 Psychostimulants and Wakefulness-Promoting Agents[19,23]

Methylphenidate: 2.5–15 mg once or twice daily
Dextroamphetamine: 2.5–15 mg once or twice daily or higher
Modafinil: 100–400 mg/day
Armodafinil: 150–250 mg/day

Box 8.11 The Role of Psychostimulants in Cancer[2,20,23,24]

Depression: Mood, apathy, psychomotor slowing
Cognitive deficits: Attention, concentration
Adjuvant analgesia: Potentiate opioid effects
Counteract sedation: Secondary to opioids
Fatigue: Weakness, hypoactivity, quality of life, mood
Appetite: Increased appetite*

* Despite the appetite suppressing effects of psychostimulants often improve energy and appetite in fatigued terminally ill patients.

than patients overall, on psychostimulants or nonamphetamine stimulants, such as modafinil.[39,40]

Summary

Fatigue is prevalent in palliative care settings and often causes significant decline in quality of life. Regular screening, assessment, education, and appropriate treatment are important to manage this distressing symptom. Given the multiple factors contributing to fatigue at the end of life, interventions should be tailored individually. A number of nonpharmacological treatment approaches have demonstrated efficacy in management of fatigue. Evidence suggests that

Table 8.1 Double-Blind, Randomized, Placebo Controlled Trials with Psychostimulants in the Treatment of Fatigue among Cancer Patients and in Palliative Care Settings

	Patient Population	Intervention	Results
Breitbart et al., 2001[32]	Double blind, RCT N = 144 Ambulatory AIDS patients with fatigue	Methylphenidate Mean dose: 49.5 mg/day Pemoline Mean dose: 98 mg/day Placebo For 6 weeks	Significant improvement in Piper Fatigue Scale Scores, VAS Fatigue Scores. Well tolerated.
Roth et al., 2010[33]	Double blind, RCT N = 32 Prostate cancer on hormonal therapy with fatigue	Methylphenidate 5–30 mg/day vs. placebo. Up to 15 mg po bid for 8 weeks	73% of patients in the intervention group reported clinically significant decrease in fatigue vs. 23% in the placebo group; 43% of men in the methylphenidate group withdrew because of cardiovascular side effects.
Lower et al., 2009[34]	Double blind RCT N = 144 patients with chemotherapy related fatigue	Dexmethylphenidate 10–50 mg/day	Compared with placebo, D-MPH treated subjects demonstrated a significant improvement in fatigue symptoms at week 8.
Bruera et al., 2006[35]	RCT, Double blind, N = 105 Cancer patients with fatigue	Methylphenidate 5 mg or placebo, q2h prn (max 4 capsules a day for 7 days)	There was no significant difference in fatigue improvement between medication and placebo arms.
Butler et al., 2007[36]	N = 68 Patients with primary or metastatic brain tumors receiving RT	D-threomethylphenidate or placebo prophylactically. Up to 15 mg po bid for 4–12 weeks.	Prophylactic use of d-threomethylphenidate did not result in an improvement in fatigue or QOL in brain tumor patients receiving RT.
Mar Fan et al., 2007[37]	N = 57 Breast cancer patients receiving adjuvant chemotherapy	d-methylphenidate up to 10 mg po bid; 20–140 days.	There were no significant differences between the randomized groups in fatigue assessment scales.
Auret et al., 2009[38]	RCT Double blind N = 50 Advanced cancer patients with fatigue in palliative care	Dexamphetamine 10 mg po bid or placebo for 8 days	There was no significant difference in fatigue improvement of quality of life between groups

(continued)

Table 8.1 (Continued)

	Patient Population	Intervention	Results
Moraska et al., 2010[39]	RCT Double blind *N* = 139 Cancer patients with fatigue	Methylphenidate 54 mg/day or placebo for 4 weeks	There was no evidence that methylphenidate, as compared with placebo, improved the primary end point of cancer-related fatigue ($P = .35$), or quality of life variables.
Bruera et al., 2013[31]	Double blind RCT Advanced cancer patients with fatigue *N* = 141	Methylphenidate 5 mg every 2 hours up to 20 mg/day or a matching placebo plus either a nursing phone intervention or a nontherapeutic control call	At the completion of the 2-week study period, there was no difference in fatigue scores between participants who had received methylphenidate and those who had received placebo. In addition to assessing the effectiveness of a pharmacologic agent, Bruera et al. have made a serious attempt to untangle the specific and the nonspecific effects of a "talking" therapy.

psychostimulants (e.g., methylphenidate) and other wakefulness agents (e.g., modafinil) can be effectively used to manage fatigue in patients with advanced disease, and therefore should be considered in the management of fatigue in palliative care settings.

References

1. Radbruch L, Strasser F, Elsner F, et al. Fatigue in palliative care patients—an EAPC approach. *Palliat Med.* 2008;22:13–32.
2. National Comprehensive Cancer Network. *NCCN Clinical Practice Guidelines in Oncology: Cancer Related Fatigue.* V.1.2013.
3. Pachman DR, Barton DL, Swetz KM, Loprinzi CL. Troublesome symptoms in cancer survivors: fatigue, insomnia, neuropathy, and pain. *J Clin Oncol.* 2012;30(30):3687–3696.
4. Portenoy RK, Thaler HT, Kornblith AB, et al. The Memorial Symptom Assessment Scale: an instrument for the evaluation of symptom prevalence, characteristics, and distress. *Eur J Cancer* 1994;30:1326–1336.
5. Piper BF, Cella D. Cancer-related fatigue: definitions and clinical subtypes. *J Natl Compr Canc Netw.* 2010;8:958–966.
6. Minton O, Stone P. A systematic review of the scales used for the measurement of cancer related fatigue. *Ann Oncol.* 2009;20:17–25.

7. Bruera E, Kuehn N, Miller MJ, et al. The Edmonton Symptom Assessment System (ESAS):A simple method for the assessment of palliative care patients. *J Palliat Care* 1991;7:6–9.
8. Cella DF, Tulsky DS, Gray G, et al. The Functional Assessment of Cancer Therapy scale: development and validation of the general measure. *J Clin Oncol.* 1993;11:570–579.
9. Mendoza TR, Wang XS, Cleeland CS, Morrissey M, Johnson BA, Wendt JK, et al. The rapid assessment of fatigue severity in cancer patients: use of the Brief Fatigue Inventory. *Cancer* 1999;85(5):1186–1196.
10. Hjermstad MJ, Fossa SD, Bjordal K, Kaasa S. Test/retest study of the European Organization for Research and Treatment of Cancer Core Quality-of-Life Questionnaire. *J Clin Oncol.* 1995;13(5):1249–1254.
11. Norcross JC, Guadagnoli E, Prochaska JO. Factor structure of the Profile of Mood States (POMS): two partial replications. *J Clin Psychol.* 1984;40(5):1270–1277.
12. Hann DM, Jacobsen PB, Azzarello LM, Martin SC, Curran SL, Fields KK, et al. Measurement of fatigue in cancer patients: development and validation of the Fatigue Symptom Inventory. *Qual Life Res.* 1998;7(4):301–310.
13. Piper BF, Dibble SL, Dodd MJ, Weiss MC, Slaughter RE, Paul SM. The revised Piper Fatigue Scale: psychometric evaluation in women with breast cancer. *Oncol Nurs Forum.* 1998;25(4):677–684.
14. Smets EM, Garssen B, Bonke B, De Haes JC. The Multidimensional Fatigue Inventory (MFI) psychometric qualities of an instrument to assess fatigue. *J Psychosom Res.* 1995;39(3):315–325.
15. Schwartz AL. The Schwartz Cancer Fatigue Scale: testing reliability and validity. *Oncol Nurs Forum.* 1998;25(4):711–717.
16. Cella D, Peterman A, Passik S, et al. Progress toward guidelines for the management of fatigue. *Oncology (Huntington)* 1998;12:369–377.
17. Yennurajalingam S, Bruera E. Palliative management of fatigue at the close of life: "It feels like my body is just worn out." *JAMA* 2007;297:295–304.
18. Stone PC, Minton O. Cancer-related fatigue. *Eur J Cancer* 2008;44:1097–1104.
19. Minton O, Richardson A, Sharpe M, et al. Drug therapy for the management of cancer-related fatigue. *Cochrane Database Syst Rev* 10.1002/14651858. CD006704.pub310.
20. Peuckmann V, Elsner F, Krumm N, et al. Pharmacological treatments for fatigue associated with palliative care. *Cochrane Database Syst Rev* 10.1002/14651858. CD006788.pub2.
21. Cramp F, Daniel J. Exercise for the management of cancer-related fatigue in adults. *Cochrane Database Syst Rev* 10.1002/14651858.CD006145.pub3.
22. Goedendorp M, Gielissen M, Verhagen C, et al. Psychosocial interventions for reducing fatigue during cancer treatment in adults. *Cochrane Database Syst Rev* 10.1002/14651858.CD006953.pub2.
23. Minton O, Richardson A, Sharpe M, et al. Psychostimulants for cancer-related fatigue: a systematic review of the literature. *J Pain Symptom Manage* 2011;41:761–767.
24. Breitbart W, Alici Y. Psychostimulants for cancer-related fatigue. *J Natl Compr Canc Netw.* 2010;8:933–942.
25. Puetz TW, Herring MP. Differential effects of exercise on cancer-related fatigue during and following treatment: a meta-analysis. *Am J Prev Med.* 2012;43(2):e1–24.

26. Jacobsen PB, Donovan KA, Vadaparampil ST, et al. Systematic review and meta-analysis of psychological and activity-based interventions for cancer-related fatigue. *Health Psychol.* 2007;26:660–667.
27. McMillan EM, et al. Exercise is an effective treatment modality for reducing cancer-related fatigue and improving physical capacity in cancer patients and survivors: a meta-analysis. *Appl Physiol Nutr Metab.* 2011 Dec;36(6):892–903. doi: 10.1139/h11-082. Epub 2011 Nov 8.
28. Bower JE, Garet D, Sternlieb B, Ganz PA, Irwin MR, Olmstead R, et al. Yoga for persistent fatigue in breast cancer survivors: a randomized controlled trial. *Cancer.* 2012;118(15):3766–3775.
29. Kangas M, Bovbjerg DH, Montgomery GH. Cancer-related fatigue: a systematic and meta-analytic review of non-pharmacological therapies for cancer patients. *Psychol Bull.* 2008;134:700–741.
30. Finnegan-John J, Molassiotis A, Richardson A, Ream E. A systematic review of complementary and alternative medicine interventions for the management of cancer-related fatigue. *Integr Cancer Ther.* 2013;12(4):276–290.
31. Bruera E, et al. Methylphenidate in the management of cancer-related fatigue. *J Clin Oncol.* 2013;31(19):2372–2373.
32. Breitbart W, Rosenfeld B, Kaim M, Funesti-Esch J. A randomized, double-blind, placebo-controlled trial of psychostimulants for the treatment of fatigue in ambulatory patients with human immunodeficiency virus disease. *Arch Intern Med.* 2001;161:411–420.
33. Roth AJ, Nelson C, Rosenfeld B. Methylphenidate for fatigue in ambulatory men with prostate cancer. *Cancer* 2010;116(21):5102–5110.
34. Lower EE, Fleishman S, Cooper A, et al. Efficacy of dexmethylphenidate for the treatment of fatigue after cancer chemotherapy: a randomized clinical trial. *J Pain Symptom Manage.* 2009;38:650–662.
35. Bruera E, Valero V, Driver L, et al. Patient-controlled methylphenidate for cancer fatigue: a double-blind, randomized, placebo-controlled trial. *J Clin Oncol.* 2006;24:2073–2078
36. Butler JM Jr, Case LD, Atkins J, et al. A phase III, double-blind, placebo-controlled prospective randomized clinical trial of d-threomethylphenidate HCl in brain tumor patients receiving radiation therapy. *Int J Radiat Oncol Biol Phys.* 2007;69:1496–1501.
37. Mar Fan HG, Clemons M, Xu W, et al. A randomised, placebo-controlled, double-blind trial of the effects of d-methylphenidate on fatigue and cognitive dysfunction in women undergoing adjuvant chemotherapy for breast cancer. *Support Care Cancer* 2008;16:577–583.
38. Auret KA, Schug SA, Bremner AP, Bulsara M. A randomized, double-blind, placebo-controlled trial assessing the impact of dexamphetamine on fatigue in patients with advanced cancer. *J Pain Symptom Manage.* 2009;37:613–621.
39. Moraska AR, Sood A, Dakhil SR, et al. Phase III, randomized, double-blind, placebo-controlled study of long-acting methylphenidate for cancer-related fatigue: North Central Cancer Treatment Group NCCTG-N05C7 trial. *J Clin Oncol.* 2010;28:3673–3679.
40. Jean-Pierre P, Morrow GR, Roscoe JA, et al. A phase 3 randomized, modafinil on cancer-related fatigue among 631 patients receiving chemotherapy: a University of Rochester Cancer Center Community Clinical Oncology Program research base study. *Cancer* 2010;116:3513–3520.

Chapter 9

Psychotherapy and Behavioral Interventions in Palliative Care

Clinicians often underestimate the potential benefits of psychotherapy and behavioral interventions for seriously medically ill patients, particularly when the patient is close to death.[1] This bias is reflected in the dearth of clinical research on psychotherapy and behavioral interventions in this population. However, a range of psychotherapeutic and behavioral interventions have been demonstrated to be quite effective and useful for patients struggling with advanced life-threatening medical illness.[1] Despite lack of evidence for prolonged survival, psychosocial interventions have been shown—through well-designed randomized controlled trials—to be effective in decreasing depressive symptoms and suffering in advanced cancer patients.[2]

Readers should refer to the *Handbook of Psychotherapy in Cancer Care*,[3] developed as part of the International Psycho-Oncology Society's (IPOS) educational strategy, edited by David Kissane and Maggie Watson, for an in-depth review of the psychotherapy interventions for cancer patients, and their caregivers (Box 9.1).

Psychotherapeutic interventions should include both the patient and family, particularly as the patient with advanced illness becomes increasingly debilitated and less capable of interaction with others. It is a time of vital importance that can often set the tone for the subsequent bereavement course.[4]

Supportive psychotherapy can be a useful treatment approach for treating distress in the terminally ill patient. Such therapy consists of active listening with supportive verbal interventions and the occasional interpretation (Box 9.2).[1]

Box 9.1 General Goals for Psychotherapy with the Dying Patient

1. Establish a bond that decreases the sense of isolation experienced with terminal illness.
2. Help the patient face death with a sense of self-worth.
3. Correct misconceptions about the past and present.
4. Integrate the present illness into a continuum of life experiences.
5. Explore issues of separation, loss, and the unknown that lies ahead.
6. Help the patient mobilize inner resources by emphasizing past strengths and supporting previously successful ways of coping.
7. Help the patient modify plans for the future, and perhaps even accept the inevitability of death.

Box 9.2 Supportive Psychotherapy with the Dying Patient: Guidelines

1. The dying patient who wishes to talk or ask questions about death should be allowed to do so freely, with the therapist maintaining an interested, interactive stance.
2. Despite the seriousness of the patient's plight, it is not necessary for the psycho-oncologist to appear overly solemn or emotionally restrained. Often it is only the psychotherapist, of all the patient's caregivers, who is comfortable enough to converse lightheartedly and allow the patient to talk about his or her life and experiences, rather than focus solely on impending death.

Traditional insight-oriented psychotherapy has had limited application among dying patients. Resolution of conflicts, through a process involving interpretation, catharsis, and enhanced insight, requires time, energy, and a commitment to an arduous psychological process. This approach may be too cumbersome for most patients nearing death. However, elements of psychodynamic therapy have an important role in all psychotherapies that can be practically applied to work with the dying, as described in the following.

Interpersonal psychotherapy has been used to treat depression and enhance coping for patients facing HIV-related disorders and in older adults with late-life depression with favorable results.[5,6] However, the applicability of interpersonal psychotherapy to patients who are imminently approaching death might be limited given the time frame of this type of intervention (Boxes 9.3–9.5).

The role of group psychotherapeutic interventions for medically ill patients has traditionally been to provide basic information, provide support, facilitate emotional expression, and teach coping skills.[1,20] The interventions listed in the following often cover a broad range of pragmatic and/or existential issues, combining psycho-education, coping skills, symptom control, support, emotional expression, and existential concerns (Boxes 9.6 and 9.7).

A relatively small, but growing, literature is developing around psychotherapy interventions for palliative care patients that are based on nontraditional,

Box 9.3 Interpersonal Psychotherapy in Patients with Advanced Illness

- Educate about the symptoms of depression.
- Place the depression in the context of present problems and solutions.
- Explore stressors in interpersonal relationships that may contribute to depression.
- Explore options for actively changing dysfunctional behavior patterns.
- Identify interpersonal problem areas, such as grief, role transition, interpersonal disputes, and interpersonal deficits.[5,6]

Box 9.4 Forms of Life Review[7–15]

- Written or taped autobiographies
- Reminiscence through storytelling of past experiences or discussion of the patient's career or life work
- Creation of family trees
- Pilgrimages
- Arts and crafts (creating a collage or drawings, poetry)
- Journal writing

Box 9.5 Use of Life Narrative and Life Review[7–15]

- Has traditionally been used for treating patients whose depression is a response to physical illness
- May be very resource intensive for patients at end stages of their illness
- Explores the meaning of physical illness in the context of one's life trajectory
- Provides patients with the opportunity to identify and re-examine past experiences and achievements in order to find meaning, resolve old conflicts, and make amends with friends and family or resolve unfinished business
- Designed to create a new perspective of dealing with illness, to increase self-esteem (by emphasizing past strengths), and to support past coping strategies
- The therapist summarizes the patient's life history and the patient's response to the illness to convey a sense that the therapist understands and knows the patient over time.
- Can bolster patients' psychological and physical well-being
- Life review has traditionally been used in the elderly population as a means of conflict resolution to help the elderly person facilitate a dignified acceptance of death. Variations of this approach are beginning to be utilized in palliative care settings.

Box 9.6 Categories of Group Psychotherapy[16]

- Patient education/psycho-education interventions[17–19]
- Supportive-expressive interventions[20–23]
- Cognitive-existential group psychotherapy[24]
- Meaning-centered group psychotherapy[25]

Box 9.7 Benefits of Group Psychotherapy in the Medically Ill[16–25]

- Time efficient and cost effective
- Highly effective in:
  1. improving quality of life;
  2. reducing psychological distress, anxiety, and depression;
  3. improving coping skills; and
  4. reducing symptoms such as pain, nausea, and vomiting
- Intervention format equal to, or even more effective than, individual psychotherapy interventions
- Provides a sense of universality; sharing a common experience and identity; a feeling of helping oneself by helping others; hopefulness fostered by seeing how others have coped successfully; and a sense of belonging to a larger group (self-transcendence, meaning, and common purpose)

alternative, spiritually based interventions that are grounded in theoretical perspectives that range from yoga, meditation, and Buddhist philosophy[26] (e.g., mindfulness-based meditation therapy), to those that are based on concepts and theories of self-transcendence.[27] Breitbart and his colleagues[25,27,28] have developed interventions for spiritual suffering in the terminally ill that focus on increasing patients' sense of meaning and purpose in life despite their illnesses. Kissane[29] has been developing an intervention aimed at targeting what he terms "demoralization syndrome" among cancer patients. Nissim and colleagues have developed an individual psychotherapy intervention that is also based on enhancing meaning in advanced cancer patients, namely, Managing Cancer and Living Meaningfully (CALM).[30] In addition, Chochinov and his collaborators[31–33] conducted work on a "dignity conserving intervention" for patients at the end of life. Palliative care practitioners have begun to recognize the importance of spiritual suffering in their patients and have begun to design interventions to address it. For more information on spiritual issues in the care of the dying, see chapter 11.

Existential therapies explore ways in which suffering can be experienced from a more positive and meaningful perspective (Box 9.8).

Initial studies examining the survival benefits of supportive-expressive psychotherapy among breast cancer patients have resulted in many more studies to replicate the findings of the initial trial. The unanimous finding of all the studies has been the positive quality of life effects of supportive expressive group psychotherapy among women with metastatic breast cancer (Box 9.9).[16,20–23]

Breitbart and colleagues[27] have applied the work of Viktor Frankl and his concepts of meaning-based psychotherapy to address spiritual suffering. Although Frankl's logotherapy was not designed for the treatment of patients with life-threatening illness, his concepts of meaning and spirituality clearly have applications in psychotherapeutic work with advanced medically ill patients, many of whom seek guidance and help in dealing with issues of sustaining meaning, hope, and understanding their illness while avoiding overt religious emphasis (Boxes 9.10–9.12).

Box 9.8 Cognitive-Existential Group Therapy[16,24]

- Developed to improve mood and mental attitude toward cancer in women with early-stage breast cancer receiving adjuvant chemotherapy
- Groups typically begin with patients sharing their experience of illness, followed by a joint focus on grief and existential concerns
- Cognitive aspects are integrated during the middle phase classes, followed by relaxation techniques (progressive muscle relaxation with guided imagery)
- Patients are encouraged to exchange phone numbers and to meet informally (e.g., over refreshments after each session) to reinforce the support gained in the therapy sessions
- Has been shown to reduce anxiety and improve family relationships

Box 9.9 Supportive-Expressive Therapy[20–23]

1. Supportive-expressive psychotherapy is based on insight-oriented psychotherapy that focuses on emotional expression, self-understanding, psychological support, and a resolution of core conflictual relationships.
2. In the terminally ill, the focus of supportive-expressive psychotherapy is frequently on the meaning of the illness, the sense of loss, the disruption in personal relationships, and the individual's sense of loss of control and competence.
3. It enables terminally ill patients to process feelings and alleviate unresolved grief.
4. It gives terminally ill patients an opportunity for reflective awareness and find meaning in past and current life experiences.

Kissane and colleagues[29] have described a syndrome of "demoralization" in the terminally ill that they propose is distinct from depression, and consists of a triad of hopelessness, loss of meaning, and existential distress expressed as a desire for death. It is associated with life-threatening medical illness, disability, bodily disfigurement, fear, loss of dignity, social isolation, and feelings of being a burden. Because of the sense of impotence and hopelessness, those with the syndrome predictably progress to a desire to die or commit suicide. Kissane and colleagues have formulated a multidisciplinary, multimodal treatment approach for demoralization syndrome (Box 9.13).[29]

Patients often experience loss of control, loss of sense of self, feeling demoralized, marginalized, and devalued by the experience of chronic illness and their failing health. Patients often draw upon what they have lost through their suffering and feel a fragmented sense of being. Terminally ill patients struggle with many existential concerns from which significant distress can arise, such as loss of meaning, value, or dignity that can diminish hope. Ensuring "dignity" in the dying process is a critical goal of palliative care.[31] Dignity is defined as the quality or state of being worthy, honored, or esteemed. In palliative care settings it

Box 9.10 The Sources of Meaning: Achieving Transcendence

1. Creativity: Work, deeds, causes
2. Experience: Nature, art, relationships
3. Attitude: The attitude one takes toward suffering and existential problems
4. Legacy: Individual, family, community history

(Adapted from Breitbart W, Appelbaum A. Cancer care, meaning-centered group psychotherapy. In: Watson M, Kissane D, eds. *Handbook of Psychotherapy*. New York: Wiley-Blackwell, 2011:137–148.)

Box 9.11 Meaning-Centered Psychotherapy: Session Topics and Themes[27]

Session #1: Concepts and Sources of Meaning
* *Introductions to Intervention and Meaning*

Session #2: Cancer and Meaning
* *Identity—Before and After Cancer Diagnosis*

Session #3: Historical Sources of Meaning
* *Life as a Living Legacy (past)*

Session #4: Historical Sources of Meaning
* *Life as a Living Legacy (present-future)*

Session #5: Attitudinal Sources of Meaning
* *Encountering Life's Limitations*

Session #6: Creative Sources of Meaning
* *Actively Engaging in Life (via creativity and responsibility)*

Session #7: Experiential Sources of Meaning
* *Connecting with Life (via: love, beauty and humor)*

Session #8: Transitions
* *Reflections and Hopes for the Future*

Box 9.12 Meaning-Centered Psychotherapy[25,27,28]

- Utilizes a mixture of didactics, discussion, and experiential exercises that focus around particular themes related to meaning and advanced cancer
- Designed to help patients with advanced cancer sustain or enhance a sense of meaning, peace, and purpose in their lives even as they approach the end of life
- Both individual meaning-centered psychotherapy and meaning-centered group psychotherapy interventions have been shown to improve spiritual well-being, meaning, quality of life, and reduce hopelessness, desire for hastened death and physical symptom distress among advanced cancer patients.

Box 9.13 Treatment Approach for Demoralization Syndrome[29]

1. Ensure continuity of care and active symptom management.
2. Ensure dignity in the dying process.
3. Explore relevant existential issues. Inquire about hope and meaning in the patient's life.
4. Utilize various types of psychotherapy (meaning-based, cognitive-behavioral, interpersonal, and family psychotherapy interventions) to help sustain a sense of meaning, limit cognitive distortions by cognitive restructuring, and maintain family relationships, as well as spiritual/religious support.
5. Use life review and narrative, with attention to spiritual issues.
6. Use pharmacotherapy for comorbid anxiety, depression, and delirium.

is essential for patients to feel that they are respected or worthy of respect despite the physical and psychological distress brought about by the illness. Maintaining feelings of physical comfort, autonomy, meaning, spiritual comfort, social connectedness, and courage are also essential components of maintaining dignity in palliative care patients. A fractured sense of dignity has been found to be associated with increased risk of hopelessness, depression, loss of will to live, and desire for hastened death.[31]

The Patient Dignity Inventory (PDI) has been developed by Chochinov and colleagues[34,35] to measure various sources of dignity related distress among patients nearing the end of life. The PDI is a valid and reliable new instrument, which could assist clinicians to routinely detect end-of-life dignity-related distress. Identifying these sources of distress is a critical step toward understanding human suffering and should help clinicians deliver quality, dignity-conserving end-of-life care. Feeling a sense of burden to others is common among dying patients. Using the PDI, a "sense of burden to others" has been demonstrated in about 60% of terminally ill patients.[34] Four variables emerged in a multiple regression analysis predicting burden to others, including hopelessness, current quality of life, depression, and level of fatigue. There was no association between sense of burden to others and actual degree of physical dependency. The lack of association between "sense of burden to others" and the degree of physical dependency suggests this perception is largely mediated through psychological and existential considerations. Strategies that target meaning and purpose, depression, and level of fatigue could lessen this source of distress and enhance quality, dignity-conserving care.[34]

The concept of dignity and the notion of dignity-conserving care offer a way of understanding how patients face advancing terminal illness, and present an approach that clinicians can use to explicitly target the maintenance of dignity as a therapeutic objective (Box 9.14).[31–33]

Most patients with advanced illness are still appropriate candidates for useful application of behavioral techniques despite physical debilitation (Boxes 9.15–9.17).

Box 9.14 Dignity Therapy Based on "Dignity Conserving Care"[31–33]

- Psychotherapeutic intervention for palliative care patients that incorporates various facets most likely to bolster the dying patient's will to live, lessen his or her desire for death or overall level of distress, and improve the quality of life
- Emphasizes "generativity" as a significant dignity theme
- Sessions are taped, transcribed, edited, and the transcription returned to the patient within 1 to 2 days.
- The creation of a tangible product that will live beyond the patient acknowledges the importance of generativity as a salient dignity issue, while also strengthening the patient's sense of purpose, meaning, and worth.
- In most instances, transcripts are left for family or loved ones, and form part of a personal legacy that the patient will have actively participated in creating and shaping.
- In a randomized controlled trial exploring the effects of dignity therapy on distress and end-of-life experience in terminally ill patients, no significant differences were noted in the distress levels before and after completion of the study in the three groups, including dignity therapy, client-centered care, or standard palliative care. For the secondary outcomes, patients reported that dignity therapy was significantly more likely to have been helpful, improve quality of life, increase sense of dignity, change how their family saw and appreciated them, and be helpful to their family.
- Dignity therapy was significantly better than client-centered care in improving spiritual well-being, and was significantly better than standard palliative care in terms of lessening sadness or depression.
- Although the ability of dignity therapy to mitigate outright distress, such as depression, desire for death, or suicidality, has yet to be proved, its benefits in terms of self-reported end-of-life experiences support its clinical application for patients nearing death.

Box 9.15 Behavior Therapy for Patients with Advanced Illness[1]

1. Take into account the mental clarity of the patient. Confusional states such as delirium interfere dramatically with a patient's ability to focus attention and thus limit the usefulness of these techniques.
2. Bear in mind that behavioral techniques can be modified so as to include even mildly cognitive impaired patients. This often involves the therapist taking a more active role by orienting the patient, creating a safe and secure environment, and evoking a conditioned response to the therapist's voice or presence.

Box 9.16 Relaxation Exercise for Anxious Patients with Advanced Illness[36]

- Usually combined with some distraction or imagery technique
- Typically the patient is first taught to relax with passive breathing, accompanied by either passive or active muscle relaxation
- Once in such a relaxed state, the patient is taught a pleasant, distracting imagery exercise.

Box 9.17 Cognitive Behavioral Therapy[37]

- May be helpful in reducing physical and emotional distress thorough a combination of behavioral interventions as described and correction of dysfunctional cognitions.
- The dysfunctional cognitions or the cognitive distortions might be related to advanced illness and its related symptoms, negative social interactions, and neurovegetative symptoms such as insomnia and fatigue.
- More useful for patients in whom prolonged survival (i.e., several months) affords the opportunity for intensive treatment

Managing Cancer and Living Meaningfully (CALM)[30] is designed as an individual therapy intended for patients with advanced disease to address the practical, relational, and existential domains of experience. Managing Cancer and Living Meaningfully is rooted in several theoretical frameworks, including relational theory, attachment theory, and existential psychotherapy. It also shares features with manualized supportive expressive, and meaning-centered group psychotherapies (Box 9.18).

Box 9.18 Managing Cancer and Living Meaningfully[30]

- The Managing Cancer and Living Meaningfully (CALM) intervention provides support and the opportunity to reflect and process thoughts and emotions evoked by the disease and its implications.
- CALM sessions cover four broad domains: (1) symptom management and communication with health care providers; (2) changes in self and relations with close others; (3) spiritual well-being or sense of meaning and purpose; and (4) issues related to advance care planning and end of life.
- Although CALM is an individual therapy, participation of the designated primary caregiver (usually the spouse or other family member) in at least one session is encouraged, allowing for more effective assessment and enhancement of family adjustment.
- Although the first session is conducted face to face, follow-up sessions may be conducted over the phone when disability or geographic distance limits the ability to attend sessions at the hospital.

Box 9.19 Family-Focused Grief Therapy[4]

The functioning of the family is screened when the patient is admitted to a service in order to identify families at risk of morbid psychosocial outcome as a result of how members relate together.

Families are then offered an intervention aimed at connecting their inherent strengths and reinforcing their capacity to cope adaptively.

It starts during palliative care of terminally ill patients and continues into bereavement.

Family-Focused Grief Therapy was developed by Kissane et al.[4] to reduce the morbid effects of grief among families at risk of poor psychosocial outcome (Box 9.19).

References

1. Rodin G. Individual psychotherapy for the patient with advanced disease. In: Chochinov HM, Breitbart W, eds. *Handbook of Psychiatry in Palliative Medicine*. New York: Oxford University Press; 2009:443–453.
2. Kissane DW. Letting go of the hope that psychotherapy prolongs cancer survival. *JCO* 2007;5689–5690.
3. Watson M, Kissane DW, eds. *Handbook of Psychotherapy in Cancer Care*. London: Wiley; 2011.
4. Kissane DW, McKenzie M, Bloch S, et al. Family focused grief therapy: a randomized, controlled trial in palliative care and bereavement. *Am J Psychiatry* 2006;163:1208–1218.
5. Markowitz JC, Kocsis JH, Fishman B, et al. Treatment of depressive symptoms in human immunodeficiency virus–positive patients. *Arch Gen Psychiatry* 1998;5:452–457.
6. Andreescu C, Reynolds CF 3rd. Late-life depression: evidence-based treatment and promising new directions for research and clinical practice. *Psychiatr Clin North Am*. 2011;34(2):335–355.
7. Neimeyer RA, Pennebaker JW, van Dyke JG. Narrative medicine: writing through bereavement. In: Chocinov HM, Breitbart W, eds. *Handbook of Psychiatry in Palliative Medicine*. New York: Oxford University Press; 2009:454–469.
8. Abiven M. Dying with dignity. *World Health Forum* 1991;12:375–381.
9. Butler RN. The life review: an interpretation of reminiscence in the aged. *Psychiatry* 1963;26:65–75.
10. Lewis MI, Butler R. Life review therapy: putting memories to work in individual and group psychotherapy. *Geriatrics* 1974;29:165–169.
11. Pickrel J. Tell me your story: using life review in counseling the terminally ill. *Death Studies* 1989;13:127–135.
12. Lichter I, Mooney J, Boyd M. Biography as therapy. *Palliat Med*. 1993;7:133–137.
13. Heiney PS. The healing power of story. *Oncol Nurs Forum* 1995;6:899–904.
14. Viederman M. The supportive relationship, the psychodynamic life narrative, and the dying patient. In: Chochinov HM, Breitbart W, eds. *Handbook of Psychiatry in Palliative Medicine*. New York: Oxford University Press; 2000:215–223.

15. Pennebaker JW, Seagal JD. Forming a story: the health benefits of narrative. *J Clin Psychol.* 1999;55:1243–1254.

16. Spiegel D, Leszcz M. Group psychotherapy and the terminally ill. In: Chocinov HM, Breitbart W, eds. *Handbook of Psychiatry in Palliative Medicine.* New York: Oxford University Press; 2009:490–503.

17. Johnson J. The effects of a patient education course on persons with a chronic illness. *Cancer Nursing* 1982;117–123.

18. Worden J, Weisman A. Preventive psychosocial intervention with newly diagnosed cancer patients. *Gen Hosp Psychiatry* 1984;6:243–249.

19. Cunningham A, Edmonds C, Hampson A, Hanson H, Hovanec M, Jenkins G, et al. A group psychoeducational program to help cancer patients cope with and combat their disease. *Advances* 1991;7:41–56.

20. Spiegel D, Bloom JR, Yalom ID. Group support for patients with metastatic cancer: a randomized prospective outcome study. *Arch Gen Psychiatry* 1981;38:527–533.

21. Spiegel D, Bloom J, Kraemer HC, et al. The effect of psychosocial treatment on survival of metastatic breast cancer patients: a randomized prospective outcome study. *Lancet* 1989;14:888–891.

22. Kissane DW, Grabsch B, Clarke DM, Smith GC, Love AW, Bloch S, et al. Supportive-expressive group therapy for women with metastatic breast cancer: survival and psychosocial outcome from a randomized controlled trial. *Psychooncology* 2007;16(4):277–286.

23. Spiegel D, Butler LD, Giese-Davis J, Koopman C, Miller E, DiMiceli S, et al. Effects of supportive-expressive group therapy on survival of patients with metastatic breast cancer: a randomized prospective trial. *Cancer* 2007;110(5):1130–1138.

24. Kissane DW, Bloch S, Smith GC, Miach P, Clarke DM, Ikin J, et al. Cognitive-existential group psychotherapy for women with primary breast cancer: a randomised controlled trial. *Psychooncology* 2003;12(6):532–546.

25. Breitbart W, Rosenfeld B, Gibson C, Pessin H, Poppito S, Nelson C, et al. Meaning-Centered Group Psychotherapy for patients with advanced cancer: a pilot randomized controlled trial. *Psycho-oncology* 2010a;(1):21–28.

26. Ando MT, Morita T, Akechi T, et al. The efficacy of mindfulness-based meditation therapy on anxiety, depression, and spirituality in Japanese patients with cancer. *J Palliat Med* 2009;12:1091–1094.

27. Breitbart W, Appelbaum A. Cancer care, meaning-centered group psychotherapy. In: Watson M, Kissane D, eds. *Handbook of Psychotherapy.* New York: Wiley-Blackwell; 2011:137–148.

28. Breitbart W, Poppito S, Rosenfeld B, Vickers AJ, Li Y, Abbey J, et al. Pilot randomized controlled trial of individual meaning-centered psychotherapy for patients with advanced cancer. *J Clin Oncol.* 2012b;30(12):1304–1309.

29. Kissane D, Clarke DM, Street AF. Demoralization syndrome: a relevant psychiatric diagnosis for palliative care. *J Palliat Care* 2001;17:12–21.

30. Nissim R, Freeman E, Lo C, Zimmermann C, Gagliese L, Rydall A, et al. A qualitative study of a brief individual psychotherapy for individuals with advanced cancer. *Palliat Med.* 2012;26(5):713–721.

31. Chochinov HM. Dignity-conserving care—a new model for palliative care: helping the patient feel valued. *JAMA.* 2002;287(17):2253–2260.

32. Chochinov HM, Hack T, Hassard T, et al. Dignity therapy: a novel psychotherapeutic intervention for patients near the end of life. *J Clin Oncol.* 2005;23:5520–5525.

33. Chochinov HM, Kristjanson LJ, Breitbart W, McClement S, Hack TF, Hassard T, et al. Effect of dignity therapy on distress and end-of-life experience in terminally ill patients: a randomised controlled trial. *Lancet Oncol*. 2011;12(8):753–762.

34. Chochinov HM, Hassard T, McClement S, Hack T, Kristjanson LJ, Harlos M, et al. The patient dignity inventory: a novel way of measuring dignity-related distress in palliative care. *J Pain Symptom Manage*. 2008;36(6):559–571.

35. Chochinov HM, McClement SE, Hack TF, McKeen NA, Rach AM, Gagnon P, et al. The Patient Dignity Inventory: applications in the oncology setting. *J Palliat Med*. 2012;15(9):998–1005.

36. Lewis EJ, Sharp DM. Relaxation and image based therapy. In: Watson M, Kissane D, eds. *Handbook of Psychotherapy in Cancer Care*. New York: Wiley-Blackwell; 2011:49–58.

37. Horne D, Watson M. Cognitive behavioral therapies in cancer care. In: Watson M, Kissane D, eds. *Handbook of Psychotherapy in Cancer Care*. New York: Wiley-Blackwell; 2011:15–26.

Chapter 10

Psychiatric and Psychological Interventions for the Control of Pain and Selected Physical Symptoms

Although the diagnosis and treatment of psychiatric disorders in the patient with advanced illness is of importance, pain and other troublesome physical symptoms must also be aggressively treated in efforts aimed at the enhancement of the patient's quality of life. These symptoms must be assessed by the psycho-oncologist concerned with the assessment and treatment of affective and other syndromes in the terminally ill population. Readers should refer to chapter 8 for an overview of the assessment and management of cancer-related fatigue. For the interested reader, a comprehensive review of pharmacological and nonpharmacological interventions for common physical symptoms encountered in the terminally ill can be found in the *Oxford Textbook of Palliative Medicine*, 3rd ed[1] and *The Handbook of Psychiatry and Palliative Medicine* (Boxes 10.1–10.3).[2]

Box 10.1 Assessment of Physical Symptoms in the Terminally Ill[3–6]

- Physical symptoms can go undetected and cause significant emotional distress. This distress often dissipates when effective management is instituted.
- It is not uncommon to observe a dramatic improvement in quality of life after adequate symptom control is achieved.
- The assessment and management of common physical symptoms must always take into account the psychosocial context and associations (e.g., more pronounced fatigue among patients with depression; increased intensity and distress owing to pain in patients with severe anxiety).
- Among cancer patients, physical symptoms such as fatigue and pain have been shown to be most prevalent. Actually, most patients experience multiple physical and psychological symptoms.[3] A survey of an outpatient cancer population has revealed more than nine concurrent symptoms.[5] Hospitalized cancer patients were shown to average more than 13 concurrent symptoms.[5] Coyle et al. reported that 70% of terminally ill patients have three or more physical symptoms other than pain.[6] This finding replicates those of earlier papers that elucidate the multiple problems facing the terminally ill patient.[3]

Box 10.2 The Goals of Symptom Assessment in Palliative Care Settings

Characterize the symptoms in terms of descriptors and impact.

Determine the likely etiologies and identification of syndromes if present.

Determine other factors that may influence the symptom expression and the degree of suffering, including physical and psychosocial comorbidities.

Reassess the nature of symptoms and the response to interventions during the course of the illness.

Box 10.3 Symptom Assessment Tools Used in Palliative Care Settings

Single-item symptom scales (numerical, visual analog, verbal category scales)[7]
Multidimensional instruments

- The Edmonton Symptom Assessment System is designed to assess symptoms in terminally ill patients, and consists of 10 visual analog scales that measure the patient's current level of pain, fatigue, nausea, depression, anxiety, drowsiness, appetite, sensation of well-being, dyspnea, and sleep.[8]
- The Memorial Symptom Assessment Scale assesses 32 physical and psychological symptoms providing information on global symptom distress, psychological symptom distress, and physical symptom distress.[9]

Pain

Adequate medical assessment and management of cancer pain is essential. The reader is directed to recent reviews by Portenoy et al.[3] and Breitbart et al.[10] for a detailed discussion of the use of behavioral, psychotherapeutic, and psychopharmacological interventions in pain control.

It is important for psycho-oncologists to be familiar with the commonly used analgesic medications in the palliative care settings in order to best assess and manage psychological aspects of pain in this patient population. Tables 10.1 and 10.2 summarize the list of pain medications commonly used in the treatment of pain from mild to severe intensity.

In brief, behavioral interventions are effective in the management of acute procedures related cancer pain, and as an adjunct in the management of chronic cancer pain (Boxes 10.4 and 10.5).[7,8]

Table 10.1 Oral Analgesics for Mild to Moderate Pain in Cancer and AIDS

Analgesic (by class)	Starting Dose (mg)	Duration (hours)	Plasma Half-Life (hrs)	Comments
Nonsteroidal Anti-inflammatory Drugs (NSAIDs)				
Aspirin	325	4–6	4–6	The standard for comparison among nonopioid analgesics
Ibuprofen	400–600	——	——	Like aspirin, can inhibit platelet function
Choline magnesium trisalicylate	700–1500	——	——	Essentially no hematological or gastrointestinal side effects
Celecoxib	100–200	11	11	Decrease dose by 50% in moderate hepatic impairment
Weaker Opioids				
Codeine	32–65	3–4	——	Metabolized to morphine, often used to suppress cough in patients at risk of pulmonary bleed
Oxycodone	5–10	3–4	——	Available as a single agent and in combination with aspirin or acetaminophen
Propoxyphene hydrochloride	65–130	4–6	——	Toxic metabolite norpropoxy accumulates with repeated dosing

(Adapted from Breitbart W, Passik S, Casper DJ, et al. Psychiatric aspects of pain in management in patients with advanced cancer and AIDS. Chochinov HMC, Breitbart W, eds. *Handbook of Psychiatry in Palliative Medicine*, 2nd ed. New York: Oxford University Press; 2009:384–416.)

Anorexia and Weight Loss

Cancer patients and their families find weight loss demoralizing, perplexing, and distressing. Weight loss and anorexia in the terminally ill patient are complex problems that can arise from a number of sources. Although most often a variety of medical factors account for the anorexia and cachexia associated with terminal illness, psychological and psychiatric factors may also play a role in the etiology of anorexia and weight loss. The most frequent such causes are anxiety, depression, and conditioned food aversions (Box 10.6).[13]

Table 10.2 Opioid Analgesics for Moderate to Severe Pain in Cancer or AIDS Patients

Analgesic	Equi-analgesic Route	Dose (mg)	Analgesic Onset (hrs)	Duration (hrs)	Plasma Half-life (hrs)	Comments
Morphine	PO	30–60*	1–1½	4–6	2–3	Standard of comparison for the opioid analgesics.
	IM, IV, SC	10	½–1	3–6		30 mg for repeat around-the-clock dosing; 60 mg for single dose or intermittent dosing.
Morphine extended release	PO	90–120	1–1½	8–12	——	Long-acting sustained release forms.
Oxycodone	PO	20–30	11	3–6	2–3	In combination with aspirin or acetaminophen, it is considered a weaker opioid; as a single agent it is comparable to the strong opioids, like morphine.
	PO (extended release)	20–40		8–12	2–3	Available in immediate-release and sustained-release preparations.
Hydromorphone	PO	7.5	½–1	3–4	2–3	Short half-life; ideal for elderly patients. Comes in suppository and injectable forms.
	IM, IV	1.5	¼–½	3–4	2–3	
Methadone	PO	20	½–1	4–8	15–30	Long half-life; tends to accumulate with initial dosing, requires careful titration. Good oral potency.
	IM, IV	10	½–1	——	15–30	
Levorphanol	PO	4	½–1½	3–6	12–16	Long half-life; requires careful dose titration in first week. Note that analgesic duration is only 4 hours.
	IM	2	½–1	3–4	12–16	
Meperidine	PO	300	½–1½	3–6	3–4	Active toxic metabolite, normeperidine, tends to accumulate (plasma half-life is 12–16 hours), especially with renal impairment and in elderly patients, causing delirium, myoclonus, and seizures.
	IM	75	½–1	3–4	3–4	
Fentanyl	TD	0.1	12–18	48–72	20–22	Transdermal patch is convenient, bypassing GI analgesia until depot is formed. Not suitable for rapid titration.
	IV	0.01		——	——	

IM, intramuscular; IV, intravenous; PO, per oral; SC, subcutaneous; TD, transdermal.
(Adapted from Breitbart W, Passik S, Casper DJ, et al. Psychiatric aspects of pain in management in patients with advanced cancer and AIDS. Chochinov HMC, Breitbart W, eds. *Handbook of Psychiatry in Palliative Medicine*, 2nd ed. New York: Oxford University Press; 2009:384–416.)

Box 10.4 Pain: Psychological Interventions[10–23]

- Hypnosis, biofeedback, and multicomponent cognitive behavioral interventions have been used to provide comfort and minimize pain in adults, children, and adolescents undergoing bone marrow aspirations, spinal taps, and other painful procedures.[10–23]
- Behavioral interventions utilized in the management of acute procedure-related pain employ the basic elements of relaxation and distraction or diversion of attention.[13,14,16]
- In chronic cancer pain, cognitive behavioral techniques are most effective when they are employed as part of a multimodal, multidisciplinary approach.[14]
- Mild to moderate levels of residual pain can be effectively managed with behavioral techniques that are quite similar to those used for anxiety, phobias, and anticipatory nausea and vomiting.

Box 10.5 Behavioral Techniques for Patients with Pain[10–18]

1. Relaxation techniques are utilized to help the patient achieve a relaxed state. Once in a relaxed state, the cancer patient with pain can use a variety of imagery techniques, including pleasant distracting imagery, transformational imagery, and dissociative imagery.
2. Transformational imagery involves the imaginative transformation of either the painful sensation itself, or the context of pain, or both. Patients can imaginatively transform a sensation of pain in their arm, for instance, into a sensation of warmth or cold. Such techniques can also be used to alter the context of the pain.
3. Dissociative imagery or dissociated somatization refers to the use of one's imagination to disconnect or dissociate from the pain experience. Specifically, patients can sometimes imagine that they leave their pain-wracked body in bed and walk about for 5 or 10 minutes pain free. Patients can also imagine that a particularly painful part of their body becomes disconnected or dissociated from the rest of them, resulting in a period of freedom from pain.
4. These techniques can provide much-needed respite from pain. Even short periods of relief from pain can break the vicious pain cycle that entraps many cancer patients.

Box 10.6 Treatment of Anorexia and Weight Loss: Guidelines and Considerations[24–41]

- Begin with the identification and correction of any reversible causes.
- Appetite may be impaired by change in taste, nausea, dysphagia, constipation, pain, and psychological distress.
- Once specific causes have been ruled out or corrected, subsequent treatment relies upon environmental manipulations. Frequent administration of favorite foods, nutritional supplements, and fluids can reverse weight loss. Dietary changes can be facilitated by referral to a dietitian.
- When poor appetite is a symptom of underlying major depression or significant anxiety, psychopharmacological interventions with antidepressants and anxiolytics are indicated.[24,26]
- The use of low-dose corticosteroids, megestrol acetate, cannabinoids, fish oil, progestational agents, olanzapine, mirtazapine, infliximab, and thalidomide, has been studied with equivocal results in management of anorexia and weight loss.[30–41]
- Practical nutritional recommendations have been reviewed by Strasser, and summarized as the eating hygiene offering guidance to cancer patients and their families in improving anorexia.[42]
- Behavioral interventions are commonly used to treat a variety of eating disorders in cancer patients, including conditioned anorexia and swallowing difficulties.
- Behavioral techniques can effectively lead to weight gain in nutritionally at-risk cancer patients.
- Conditioned difficulties with eating, swallowing, and nausea have been managed successfully with systematic desensitization.
- Hypnosis has been utilized in children with cancer, resulting in improved appetite and weight gain.

Nausea and Vomiting

Approximately 50% of patients with advanced cancer experience nausea and vomiting during the course of their illness (Box 10.7).[24,43]

During the course of chemotherapy, many patients become sensitized to the treatment, develop phobic-like reactions, and even develop conditioned responses to stimuli in the hospital setting. As a result of being conditioned by the experience of profound nausea and vomiting secondary to highly emetic chemotherapy agents, patients report being nauseated in anticipation of treatment (Boxes 10.8 and 10.9).

Nausea and vomiting in palliative care settings is common and distressing. Although psycho-oncologists most commonly encounter and asked to manage

Box 10.7 Common Causes of Nausea and Vomiting in Cancer Patients[3,24]

- Radiation
- Medications
- Toxins
- Metabolic derangements
- Hepatic failure
- Renal failure
- Obstruction of the gastrointestinal tract
- Autonomic neuropathy
- Chemotherapy
- Intracranial neoplasms or other intracranial lesions
- Anxiety disorders
- Conditioned responses

Box 10.8 Factors That Increase the Likelihood of Developing Anticipatory Nausea and Vomiting[44–46]

1. Severity of post-treatment nausea and vomiting (high density, duration, and frequency)
2. A pattern of increasing nausea and vomiting
3. Receiving highly emetic drugs (cis-platinum) or combinations of chemotherapies

anticipatory nausea and vomiting, it is important to be familiar with other sources of nausea and vomiting in palliative care settings. Radiation therapy, opioids, intestinal obstruction, and increased intracranial pressure are other causes of nausea and vomiting that require an interdisciplinary approach with involvement of oncology, palliative care, and psychiatry teams to vigorously provide relief of this distressing symptom at the end of life.

Insomnia

Insomnia, defined as insufficient duration or poor quality of sleep, is common among cancer patients at all stages of the illness. Difficulty falling asleep, staying asleep, or nonrestorative sleep are reported in 25% to 60% of cancer patients. Pain, delirium, depression, anxiety disorders, poor sleep hygiene,

Box 10.9 Psychiatric and Psychological Treatment of Anticipatory Nausea and Vomiting[44,47–50]

- Given the relationship between intensity of postchemotherapy nausea and vomiting and the development of anticipatory nausea and vomiting (ANV), the efficacy of antiemetic regimens in the management of these symptoms becomes increasingly important. Antiemetic drugs are the mainstay of managing chemotherapy-induced nausea and vomiting in patients with advanced disease.
- Antipsychotic medications, anticholinergic agents, antihistamines, corticosteroids, prokinetic drugs, cannabinoids, 5-HT antagonists, and benzodiazepines are the main classes of antiemetic drugs that have been used effectively in the management of nausea and vomiting in terminally ill cancer patients.
- Rapid-onset, short-acting benzodiazepines are helpful in controlling ANV once it has developed. Alprazolam has been shown to be clinically effective in reducing ANV in doses of 0.25 to 0.5 mg tid to qid, given for 1 to 2 days before chemotherapy.
- Conditioned nausea and vomiting is often quite responsive to relaxation training, guided imagery, video game distraction (in children), and other behavioral techniques.
- Chemotherapy nurses trained in these techniques can remarkably improve the quality of life in chemotherapy patients.

circadian rhythm disturbances, in cancer and cancer treatments have all been reported to contribute to sleep disturbances in palliative care settings. Psycho-oncologists should be familiar with common etiologies, assessment, and pharmacological and nonpharmacological management of insomnia in the terminally ill (Box 10.10).[52]

Box 10.10 Pharmacological and Nonpharmacological Management of Insomnia[52–54]

- Behavioral interventions have been successfully applied to the treatment of insomnia in cancer patients. Such techniques include progressive muscle relaxation training and relaxation and imagery techniques.
- Occasionally, sleep disturbance in cancer patients may be caused by a concomitant psychiatric disorder such as depression or delirium. Obviously, specific treatment for the underlying disorder is the preferred approach in these cases.
- Pharmacotherapy utilizing benzodiazepines, antidepressants, low-dose antipsychotics, and nonbenzodiazepine sedative hypnotics may also be indicated when sleep disturbance is caused by medication side effects or some other organic etiology.

References

1. Hanks G, Cherny N, Christakis N, eds. *Oxford Textbook of Palliative Medicine*, 4th ed. New York: Oxford University Press; 2010.
2. Chochinov HMC, Breitbart W, eds. *Handbook of Psychiatry in Palliative Medicine*, 2nd ed. New York: Oxford University Press; 2009.
3. Portenoy RK, El Osta B, Bruera E. Physical symptom management in the terminally ill. In: Chochinov HMC, Breitbart W, eds. *Handbook of Psychiatry in Palliative Medicine*, 2nd ed. New York: Oxford University Press; 2009:355–383.
4. Bruera E, Neumann C, Brenneis C., et al. Frequency of symptom distress and poor prognostic indicators in palliative cancer patients admitted to a tertiary palliative care unit, hospices, and acute care hospitals. *J Palliative Care* 2000;16:16–21.
5. Portenoy RK, Thaler HT, Kornblith AB, et al. Symptom prevalence, characteristics, and distress in a cancer population. *Qual Life Res*. 1994;3:183–189.
6. Coyle N, Adelhardt J, Foley KM, Portenoy RK. Character of terminal illness in the advanced cancer patient: pain and other symptoms during the last four weeks of life. *J Pain Symptom Manage*. 1990;5:83–93.
7. El Osta B, Braiteh F, Palmer J, Reddy SK, Bruera E. Characteristics, findings, and outcomes of palliative care inpatient consultations at a comprehensive cancer center. *J Palliative Med*. 2007;10(4):948–955.
8. Bruera E, Kuehn N, et al. The Edmonton Symptom Assessment System: a simple method for the assessment of palliative care patients. *J Palliative Care* 1991;7:6–9.
9. Portenoy RK, Thaler HT, Kornblith AS, et al. The Memorial Symptom Assessment Scale: an instrument for the evaluation of symptom prevalence, characteristics, and distress. *Eur J Cancer* 1994;30A:1326–1336.
10. Breitbart W, Passik S, Casper DJ, et al. Psychiatric aspects of pain in management in patients with advanced cancer and AIDS. In: Chochinov HMC, Breitbart W, eds. *Handbook of Psychiatry in Palliative Medicine*, 2nd ed. New York: Oxford University Press; 2009:384–416.
11. Spiegel D, Bloom JR. Group therapy and hypnosis reduce metastatic breast carcinoma pain. *Psychosom Med*. 1983;4:33–39.
12. Syrajala K, Cummings C, Donaldson G. Hypnosis or cognitive behavioral training for the reduction of pain and nausea during cancer treatment: a controlled trial. *Pain* 1992;48:137–146.
13. Tan SY, Leucht CA. Cognitive-behavioral therapy for clinical pain control: a 15 year update and its relationship to hypnosis. *Int J Clin Exp Hypn*. 1997;45(4):396–416.
14. Horne D, Watson M. Cognitive behavioral therapies in cancer care. In: Watson M, Kissane D, eds. *Handbook of Psychotherapy in Cancer Care*. New York: Wiley-Blackwell; 2011:15–26.
15. Cleeland CS. Nonpharmacologic management of cancer pain. *J Pain Symptom Manage*. 1987;2:523–528.
16. Loscalzo M, Jacobsen PB. Practical behavioral approaches to the effective management of pain and distress. *J Psychosoc Oncol*. 1990;8:139–169.
17. Montgomery GH, DuHamel KN, Redd WH. A meta-analysis of hypnotically induced analgesia: how effective is hypnosis? *Int J Clin Exp Hypn*. 2000;48(2):138–153.

18. Rajasekaran M, Edmonds PM, Higginson IL. Systematic review of hypnotherapy for treating symptoms in terminally ill adult cancer patients. *Palliat Med.* 2005;19(5):418–426.

19. Montgomery GH, Weltz CR, Seltz M, Bovbjerg DH. Brief presurgery hypnosis reduces distress and pain in excisional breast biopsy patients. *Int J Clin Exp Hypn.* 2002;50(1):17–32.

20. Keefe FJ, Ahles TA, Sutton L, et al. Partner-guided cancer pain management at the end of life: a preliminary study. *J Pain Symptom Manage.* 2005;29(3):263–272.

21. Hilgard JR, LeBaron S. Relief of anxiety and pain in children and adolescents with cancer: quantitative measures and clinical observations. *Int J Clin Exp Hypn.* 1982;30(4):417–442.

22. Jay SM, Elliott CH, Varni JW. Acute and chronic pain in adults and children with cancer. *J Consult Clin Psychol.* 1986;54:601–607.

23. Kellerman J, Zeltzer L, Ellenberg L, Dash J. Adolescents with cancer: Hypnosis for the reduction of the acute pain and anxiety associated with medical procedures. *Journal of Adolescents Health Care* 1983;4:85–90.

24. McClement SE, et al. Eating issues in palliative cancer patients. In: Chochinov HMC, Breitbart W, eds. *Handbook of Psychiatry in Palliative Medicine*, 2nd ed. New York: Oxford University Press; 2009:417–427.

25. Bruera E, MacDonald N. Nutrition in patients with advanced cancer: an update and review of our experience. *J Pain Sympt Manage.* 1991;6:352–359.

26. Del Fabbro E, Dalal S, Bruera E. Symptom control in palliative care part II: cachexia, anorexia and fatigue. *J Palliative Med.* 2006;9(2):409–421.

27. Lesko LM. Psychosocial issues in the diagnosis and management of cancer cachexia and anorexia. *Nutrition.*1989;5(2):114–116.

28. Dixon J. Effect of nursing interventions on nutritional and performance status in cancer patients. *Nurs Res.* 1984;33(6):330–335.

29. Campbell DF, Dixon JK, Sanderford LD, Denicola MA. Relaxation: its effect on the nutritional status and performance status of clients with cancer. *J Am Diet Assoc.* 1984;84(2):201–204.

30. Schell H. Adrenal corticosteroid therapy in far advanced cancer. *Geriatrics* 1972;27:131–141.

31. Willox JC, et al. Prednisolone as an appetite stimulant in patients with cancer. *Br Med J* 1984;200:273–288.

32. Bruera E, et al. A controlled trial of megestrol acetate on appetite, caloric intake, nutritional status, and other symptoms in patients with advanced cancer. *Cancer* 1990;66:1279–1282.

33. Loprinzi CL, et al. Randomized comparison of megestrol acetate versus dexamethasone versus fluoxymestrone for the treatment of cancer anorexia/cachexia. *J Clin Oncol.* 1999;17:3229–3306.

34. Pascual Lopez A, Roque I, Fuguls M, Urrutia C, et al. Systematic review of megestrol acetate in the treatment of anorexia-cachexia syndrome. *J Pain Symptom Manage.* 2004;27:360–369.

35. Cannabis in cachexia study group, Strasser F, Luftner D, Possinger K, et al. Comparison of orally administered cannabis extract and delta-9-hydrocannabinol in treating patients with cancer-related anorexia-cachexia syndrome: a multicenter, phase III, randomized, double-blind, placebo-controlled clinical trial. *J Clin Oncol.* 2006;24:3394–3400.

36. Gordon JN, Trebble TM, Ellis RD, Duncan HD, Johns T, Goggin PM. Thalidomide in the treatment of cancer cachexia: a randomized placebo controlled trial. *Gut* 2005;54:540–545.

37. Jatoi A, Jett JR, Sloan J, et al. A pilot study on safety and pharmacokinetics of infliximab for the cancer anorexia/weight loss syndrome in non small cell lung cancer patients. *Support Care Cancer* 2004;12:859–863.

38. Persson C, Glimelius B, Ronalid J, Nygren P. Impact of fish oil and melatonin on cachexia in patients with advanced gastrointestinal cancer: a randomized pilot study. *Nutrition* 2005;21:170–178.

39. Bruera E, Strasser F, Palmer JL, et al. Effect of fish oil on appetite and other symptoms in patients with advanced cancer and anorexia/cachexia: a double blind placebo controlled study. *J Clin Oncol.* 2003;21:129–134.

40. Jatoi A, Rowland K, Loprinzi CL, et al. An eicosapentaenoic acid supplement versus megestrol acetate versus both for patients with cancer-associated wasting. *J Clin Oncol.* 2004;22:2469–2476.

41. Davis MP, Khawam E, Pozuelo L, Lagman R. Management of symptoms associated with advanced cancer: olanzapine and mirtazapine. A WHO project. *Expert Rev Anticancer Ther.* 2002;2:365–376.

42. Strasser R. Eating-related disorders in patients with advanced cancer. *Support Care Cancer* 2003;11(1):11–20.

43. Dalal S, Del Fabbro E, Bruera E. Symptom control in palliative care. Part I: Oncology as a paradigmatic example. *J Palliative Med.* 2006;9(2):389–390.

44. Ramchandran K, Von Roenn JH. Nausea and vomiting. In: Holland J, Breitbart W, Jacobsen P, eds. *Psycho-Oncology*, 2nd ed. New York: Oxford University Press; 2010:229–235.

45. Osoba D, Zee B, Pater J, Warr D, et al. Determinants of post chemotherapy nausea vomiting in patients with cancer. *J Clin Oncol.* 1997;15:116–123.

46. Warr DG. Chemotherapy and cancer related nausea and vomiting. *Curr Oncol.* 2008;15 (suppl 1):S4–S9.

47. Figueroa-Moseley C, Jean Pierre P, Roscose J. Behavioral interventions in treating anticipatory nausea and vomiting. *J Natl Compr Cancer Network* 2007;5:44–50.

48. Greenberg DB, Surman OS, Clarke J, et al. Alprazolam for phobic nausea and vomiting related to cancer chemotherapy. *Cancer Treatment Reports* 1987;71, 549–550.

49. Flake ZA, Scalley RD, Bailey AG. Practical selection of antiemetics. *Am Fam Physician* 2004;69:1169–1174.

50. Lindlet C, Blower P. Oral serotonin tye 3 receptor antagonists for prevention of chemotherapy induced emesis. *Am J Health Syst Pharm.* 2000;57:1685–1697.

51. Mannix K. Palliation of nausea and vomiting in malignancy. *Clin Med.* 2006;6:144–147.

52. Yue HJ, Dimsdale JE. Sleep and cancer. In: Holland J, Breitbart W, Jacobsen P, eds. *Psycho-Oncology*, 2nd ed. New York: Oxford University Press; 2010:258–269.

53. Fiorentino L, Ancoli-Israel S. Insomnia and its treatment in women with breast cancer. *Sleep Med Rev.* 2006;10(6):419–429.

54. Espie CA, Fleming L, Cassidy J, et al. Randomized controlled clinical effectiveness trial of cognitive behavior therapy compared with treatment as usual for persistent insomnia in patients with cancer. *J Clin Oncol.* 2008;30:26(28):4651–4658.

Chapter 11

Spiritual and Existential Issues in the Care of the Dying

The Spiritual Domain of Care

Spirituality is an important part in the lives of patients with serious illness. Medical professionals, patients, and patients' families agree that addressing spiritual domains of palliative care is a priority at the end of life. Despite the paucity of data in this field there are convincing data that support the essential role of spirituality in people's lives, especially in the context of terminal illness.[1] An Institute of Medicine (IOM) report identified spiritual well-being as one of the most important influences on quality of life at the end of life.[2] Guidelines from a number of professional organizations, including the American College of Physicians, the Association of the American Medical Colleges, and the Joint Commission on Healthcare Accreditation recognize the need of spiritual care and require that spiritual care be available to patients (Boxes 11.1–11.4).[1,3,4]

Spirituality in Palliative Care: Communication and Assessment

The majority of studies demonstrate that patients welcome discussions about spirituality.[8,10,11] Therefore, although all the preceding factors may act as obstacles, discussions about spirituality and spiritual issues should not be avoided. Rather, such discussions may simply require more consideration on the part of the provider to overcome barriers. Several factors inhibit effective communication with patients about spirituality in the palliative care setting (Boxes 11.5–11.8).[12–15]

Terminally patients may experience a number of spiritual issues, including but not limited to lack of meaning, guilt, shame, hopelessness, loss of dignity, loneliness, anger toward God, abandonment by God, feeling out of control, grief, and spiritual suffering.

Assessing a patient's spiritual beliefs, assessing the importance of spirituality in his or her life, exploring whether he or she belongs to a spiritual community, and offering chaplaincy referral or connection with the patient's religious or spiritual leaders comprise essential components of a spiritual assessment.

Box 11.1 Domains of Quality Palliative Care from the Professional Perspective[2]

1. Overall quality of life
2. Physical well-being and functioning
3. Psychosocial well-being and functioning
4. Spiritual well-being
5. Patient perception of care
6. Family well-being and functioning

Box 11.2 Domains of Quality Palliative Care from the Patient Perspective[5]

1. Receiving adequate pain and symptom control
2. Avoiding inappropriate prolongation of dying
3. Achieving a sense of spiritual peace
4. Relieving burden
5. Strengthening relationships with loved ones

Box 11.3 Most Important Needs of Cancer Patients[6]

- Overcoming fear (51%)
- Finding hope (41%)
- Finding meaning in life (40%)
- Finding peace of mind (43%)
- Finding spiritual resources (39%)

Although there are several methods for taking a spiritual history, health care providers can structure the interview using FICA (Faith/Belief/Meaning, Importance and Influence, Community, and Address/Action in Care) (Boxes 11.9 and 11.10).[20]

Health care providers can obtain a detailed spiritual assessment in order to elicit beliefs that are relevant to good patient care. Yet this discussion should not be limited to one occasion. Instead it is the beginning of a dialogue that continues throughout a patient's care and communicates to the patient that his or her concerns will be met in a supportive and respectful manner.[21] Providers can offer great comfort to patients by a compassionate presence, reflective listening, offering empathetic responses, and inquiry about spiritual values and beliefs, life review, and continued presence in addition to referral to chaplaincy.[22]

Box 11.4 Definitions of Spirituality, Faith, and Meaning in Life

Spirituality

Spirituality is defined as a relationship outside of one's self. It is defined in terms of personal views and behaviors that express a sense of relatedness to a transcendent dimension or something greater than one's self. Spirituality is expressed in an individual's search for ultimate meaning through participation in religion and/or belief in God, family, naturalism, rationalism humanism, and the arts.[1,7,8]

Faith

A belief in a higher transcendent power, not necessarily identified as God, and not necessarily through participation in the rituals or beliefs of a specific organized religion. The relationship and connectedness to this power, or spirit, is an essential component of the spiritual experience and is related to the concept of meaning.

Meaning (or having a sense that one's life has meaning)

The conviction that one is fulfilling a unique role and purpose in a life that comes with a responsibility to live to one's full potential as a human being. In so doing, one is able to achieve a sense of peace, contentment, or even transcendence through connectedness with something greater than one's self[9]

The "faith" component of spirituality is most often associated with religion and religious belief, whereas the "meaning" component of spirituality appears to be a more universal concept that can exist in religious or nonreligious individuals.

Box 11.5 Barriers to Effective Communication with Patients about Spirituality

- The great discrepancy between physicians and patients on such issues as belief in God, belief in an afterlife, regular prayer, and feeling close to God. Physicians endorse such beliefs or practices less than half as often as patients.[16]
- Lack of time on the part of the provider
- Lack of training for physicians in this area
- Fear of health care provider projecting own beliefs onto the patient
- Concerns about patient autonomy
- A feeling among providers that these discussions are inappropriate, as they are outside of their area of expertise or intrusive to the patient's privacy[13–15]

Box 11.6 Important Domains of Knowledge for Effective Communication about Spirituality

1. A basic knowledge of common spiritual concerns and sources of spiritual pain for patients
2. The principles and beliefs of the major religions common to the patient populations one treats
3. Basic clinical communication skills, such as active and empathetic listening, with an ability to identify and highlight spiritually relevant issues
4. The ability to remain present while patients struggle with spiritual issues in light of their mortality.[17] This final domain is often the most trying, especially for clinicians early in their career.

Box 11.7 The American Academy of Hospice and Palliative Medicine Guidelines for Communicating about Spiritual Issues[1,17,18]

1. Recognize that every patient is an individual and has a unique belief system that should be honored and respected.
2. A patient's spiritual views may or may not incorporate religious beliefs, as spirituality is considered the more inclusive category. Therefore, initial discussions should focus on broad spiritual issues, followed by more specific religious beliefs when appropriate.
3. Caregivers should maintain appropriate boundaries and avoid discussions of their own religious beliefs, as this is usually not relevant.
4. Fostering hope and integrating meaning into a patient's life are more important aspects of providing spiritual healing than any adherence to a particular belief system or religious affiliation.

Box 11.8 Communication Strategies for Eliciting Spiritual Concerns

- Use open-ended questions.
- Ask patients to say more about a subject as a follow-up question.
- Acknowledge and normalize patient concerns.
- Use empathetic comments in response to patient concerns, and inquire about patient's emotions around these issues.[19]

Researchers interested in assessment of spirituality and related constructs commonly utilize one or more of the measures highlighted in Box 11.11.

Spirituality in Palliative Care: Impact and Intervention

There has been great interest in spirituality, faith, and religious beliefs with regard to their impact on health outcomes and their role in palliative care (Box 11.12).[15,25–28]

Box 11.9 Taking a Spiritual History[1,20]

Faith or beliefs

What is your faith or belief?

What things do you believe in that give meaning to life?

Do you consider yourself spiritual or religious?

Importance and influence

Is it important in your life?

What influence does it have on how you take care of yourself?

How have your beliefs influenced your behavior during this illness?

Community

Are you part of a spiritual or religious community?

Are they important to you as a source of support?

Is there a person or group of people whom you really love or who is/are really important to you?

Address

How would you like me, your health care provider, to address these issues in your care?

Box 11.10 Other Recommended Questions to Ask When Taking a Spiritual History

- Do your religious or spiritual beliefs provide comfort and support or cause stress?
- Could your spiritual or religious beliefs influence your medical decisions?
- Do you have beliefs that might conflict with your medical care?
- What are your spiritual needs?

Box 11.11 Research Measures Commonly Utilized to Assess Aspects of Spirituality[1,23,24]

Measures of Spirituality and Religion

FACIT Spiritual Well-Being Scale (FACITSWBS)—Meaning and Faith Subscales

Royal Free Spirituality Scale (RFSS)

Daily Spiritual Experiences Scale (DSES)

Measures of Religious Beliefs, Practices, Support, Coping

Spiritual Beliefs Inventory (SBI-15)

Religious Orientation Scale (ROS)

Private Religious Practices Scale (RPS)

Religious Support (Long and Short Forms)

RCOPE and Brief RCOPE

Measures of Spirituality and Meaning

Post-Traumatic Growth Inventory

FACIT-SWB Meaning Subscale

Purpose in Life Scale (PIL)

Box 11.12 Impact of Spirituality, Religion, and Faith in Palliative Care

- Some researchers theorize that religious beliefs may play a role in helping patients construct meaning out of the suffering inherent to illness, in turn facilitating acceptance of their situation.[28]
- Recent studies have found that religion and spirituality generally play a positive role in patients coping with illnesses such as HIV and cancer.[21,29,30]
- Several studies[21,31,32] demonstrate a central role for spiritual well-being and meaning as a buffer against depression, hopelessness, and desire for hastened death among advanced cancer patients.
- A 2013 study by Balboni and colleagues[33] demonstrated that patients reporting high spiritual support from religious communities were less likely to receive hospice, and more likely to receive aggressive end-of-life measures, and more likely to die in an intensive care unit. Among patients well-supported by religious communities, receiving spiritual support from the medical team was associated with higher rates of hospice use and fewer aggressive interventions. This study highlights the importance integrating spiritual care as a key component of the end of life medical care guidelines. Spiritual care and end-of-life discussions by the medical team may reduce aggressive treatment and ICU deaths, and increase the use of hospice care services among those patients.

These findings are significant in the face of what we have come to learn about the consequences of depression and hopelessness in palliative care patients. Depression and hopelessness are associated with poorer survival in cancer patients[34] as well as dramatically higher rates of suicide, suicidal ideation, desire for hastened death, and interest in physician-assisted suicide (see chapter 6).[31,35–37]

Such findings point to the need for the development of interventions in palliative patients that address depression, hopelessness, loss of meaning, desire for death, and what many practitioners[38] refer to as "spiritual suffering" (see chapter 9) (Boxes 11.13 and 11.14).

Box 11.13 Approach for the Treatment of Spiritual Suffering[*,38]

1. Control physical symptoms.
2. Provide a supportive presence.
3. Encourage life review to assist in recognizing purpose value and meaning.
4. Explore guilt, remorse, forgiveness, reconciliation.
5. Facilitate religious expression.
6. Reframe goals.
7. Encourage meditative practices.
8. Focus on healing rather than cure.

* This intervention emphasizes the facilitation of religious expression and confession. Although this is useful *for* certain patients, it is not applicable to all patients.

Box 11.14 Spiritual Issues in Palliative Care: Conclusions[1,39]

- Psycho-oncologists should be aware of the importance of spirituality as a tool for coping with a life-threatening disease and managing the stressors that can occur as a consequence of advanced disease.
- By understanding and respecting their beliefs, clinicians may allow their patients to believe in their own abilities to cope.
- Psycho-oncologists should seek both specialized training, as well as referrals to appropriate sources, in order to help patients deal more effectively with the often complicated and painful spiritual issues that arise as a consequence of serious illness.
- It is essential to effectively utilize an interdisciplinary team approach that incorporates members of pastoral care services. Referrals to chaplains should be approached as referrals to any other specialist, and are an essential part of comprehensive care.[39]

Existential Issues in Palliative Care

As human beings (homo sapiens—sapient meaning wise or capable of higher thought), we—as opposed to other creatures—are confronted by three fundamental existential questions: Where did I come from? Why am I here? Where am I going (i.e., what lies beyond death)? Vicktor Frankl felt there were three inevitable existential problems.[9] He termed these the tragic triad: suffering, death, and existential guilt (unlike our common understanding of guilt, Frankl emphasized guilt as a force that calls one to live up to one's authentic potential). Existential writers conceptualize four basic existential concerns, described in Box 11.15.[40]

Box 11.15 Basic Existential Concerns

- *Death*—death anxiety, the limitations of life, nonexistence, mortality, and finiteness; life limitations
- *Freedom*—absence of external structure, existential groundlessness, the ability to respond to life or "responsibility," free choice, awareness of personal agency, and tyranny of freedom
- *Isolation*—existential isolation, not intrapersonal or interpersonal, transcendence, and connection to something greater than ourselves
- *Meaninglessness*—the will, search, and creation of meaning in order to bear one's life, purpose, values, and contributions to a greater whole

Table 11.1 Common Manifestations of Existential Distress in Palliative Care[41]

Common Forms of Existential Distress	Manifestations
Existential angst—"death anxiety"	Feeling of "being strangled to death" (angst from Latin "*angere*," meaning "to squeeze," or "to strangle")
Existential guilt Call to take ownership of one's life Responding less to others Responding more to one's self	Expressed as not having lived to the fullest potential; feel accountable for mistakes; desire to correct a wrong
Existential suffering Profound feeling of absence (being away) from presence and abundance of life	Question value of continued existence; gradually disconnect from life; isolation, loss of sense of self; present multidimensional distress: physically—fatigue, pain, nausea emotionally—sadness, worry, anxiety, loss of dignity, being a burden spiritually—despair, loneliness

Adapted from Kissane DW, Poppito S. Death and dying. In: Blumenfield M, Strain JJ, eds. *Psychosomatic Medicine*. Philadelphia: Lippincott Williams & Wilkins; 2006:671–694.

Patients diagnosed with terminal cancer often confront these universal existential issues. Existential concerns are intrinsic to the human experience of facing mortality in palliative care settings. Therefore, psycho-oncologists must be familiar with these existential concerns, their manifestations, and approaches to deal with existential issues. Psycho-oncologists can actively help dying patients engage in existential themes of presence, mystery, and transcendence and promote authentic self-awareness, responsibility, and meaning (Table 11.1).[41]

Optimal palliative care includes the use of proper medical and therapeutic interventions, as well as an existential phenomenological approach to deal with existential distress at the end of life (Table 11.2).

As a part of the palliative care team, the psycho-oncologist plays a critical role in identifying and addressing existential concerns of dying patients. Psycho-oncologists may not only help patients cope with life's limitations, but also encourage patients to discover meaning in anxiety, guilt, and suffering. Psycho-oncologists have the unique ability to use a variety of psychotherapeutic interventions to alleviate existential distress in palliative care settings. Cognitive therapies to help patients and families modify their appraisal of their lives with terminal illness, known as cognitive restructuring, life review techniques to facilitate a constructive reappraisal of life events, dignity conserving therapies, and meaning-centered therapies have been shown to effectively reduce existential distress in this patient population.[42–44] Readers should refer to chapter 10 for a review of the psychotherapy interventions.

Table 11.2 Approaches to Existential Issues in the Terminally Ill[41]

Existential Concern	Form of Existential Distress	Symptoms Experienced	Approaches
Death	Death anxiety	Fears of process of dying or state of being dead	Psychoeducational therapy, cognitive behavioral therapy, existential psychotherapy
Loss	Complicated grief	Depressive disorders	Supportive psychotherapy, grief therapy, interpersonal psychotherapy
Existential			
Isolation	Loneliness	Feeling disconnected	Interpersonal psychotherapy, Family-focused grief therapy, supportive group therapy, meaning-centered therapy
Loss of meaning	Despair Hopelessness Desire for hastened death	Loss of identity Meaninglessness	Existential psychotherapy, meaning-centered therapy, narrative and dignity-conserving therapies
Freedom	Loss of control	Angst at loss of control, obsessional behaviors, indecisive	Supportive psychotherapy, interpersonal psychotherapy, psychodynamic therapy,
Dignity	Demoralization Desire for hastened death	Shame, body image, fear of being a burden	Supportive psychotherapy, grief therapy, narrative and dignity-conserving therapies

Adapted from Kissane DW, Poppito S. Death and dying. In: Blumenfield M, Strain JJ, eds. *Psychosomatic Medicine*. Philadelphia: Lippincott Williams & Wilkins; 2006:671–694.

References

1. Puchalski CM. Spiritual issues in palliative care. In: Chochinov HMC, Breitbart W, eds. *Handbook of Psychiatry in Palliative Medicine*, 2nd ed. New York: Oxford University Press; 2009:341–351.
2. Field M, Cassel C, eds. *Approaching Death: Improving Care at the End of Life.* Washington, DC: National Academy Press; 1997.
3. Puchalski CM, Anderson MB, Lo B, et al. *The development and dissemination of physician/patient guidelines on ethical parameters for incorporating spirituality in to medical education and health care report.* AAMC Consensus Conference, 2004.

4. Lo B, Quill T, Tulsky J. Discussing palliative care with patients. ACP-ASIM end of life care consensus panel. *Ann Intern Med.* 1999;130:744–749.
5. Singer P, Martin DK, Kelner M. Quality end-of-life care: patients' perspectives. *JAMA.* 1999;281:163–168.
6. Moadel A, Morgan C, Fatone A, et al. Seeking meaning and hope: Self-reported spiritual and existential needs among an ethnically diverse cancer patient population. *Psycho-oncology* 1999;8:1428–1431.
7. Sulmasy DP. A biopsychosocial spiritual model for the care of patients at the end of life. *Gerontologist* 2002;42:24–33.
8. King DE, Bushwick B. Beliefs and attitudes of hospital inpatients about faith, healing, and prayer. *J Fam Pract.* 1994;39:349–352.
9. Frankl VF. *Man's Search for Meaning*, 4th ed. Boston: Beacon Press; 1959/1992.
10. Anderson JM, Anderson LJ, Felsenthal G. Pastoral needs for support within an inpatient rehabilitation unit. *Arch Phys Medicine Rehabil.* 1993;74:574–578.
11. Maugans TA. The SPIRITual history. *Arch Fam Med.* 1996;5:11–16.
12. Clayton CL. Barriers, boundaries, & blessings: ethical issues in physicians' spiritual involvement with patients. *Med Humanities Rpt*, 2000;21:234–256.
13. Ellis M, Vinson D, Ewigman B. Addressing spiritual concerns of patients: family physicians' attitudes and practices. *J Fam Pract* 1999;48:105–109.
14. Post SG, Puchalski CM, Larson DB. Physicians and patient spirituality: professional boundaries, competency, and ethics. *Ann Intern Med.* 2000;132:578–583.
15. Sloan RP, Bagiella E, Powell T. Religion, spirituality, and medicine. *Lancet* 1999;353:664–667.
16. Maugans TA, Wadland WC. Religion and family medicine: a survey of physicians and patients. *J Fam Pract.* 1991;32:210–213.
17. Storey P, Knight C. UNIPAC Two: alleviating psychological and spiritual pain in the terminally ill. *American Academy of Hospice and Palliative Medicine.* Dubuque, IA: Kendall/Hunt; 2001.
18. Doyle D. Have we looked beyond the physical and psychosocial? *J Pain Symptom Manage.* 1992;7:302–311.
19. Lo B, Kates LW, Ruston D, et al. Responding to requests regarding prayer and religious ceremonies by patients near the end of life and their families. *J Palliative Med.* 2003;3:409–415.
20. Puchalski C, Romer AL. Taking a spiritual history allows clinicians to understand patients more fully. *J Palliative Med.* 2000;3:129–137.
21. Nelson CJ, Rosenfeld B, Breitbart W, et al. Spirituality, religion, and depression in the terminally ill. *Psychosomatics* 2002;43:213–220.
22. Breitbart W. The spiritual domain of palliative care: who should be "spiritual care professionals" *Palliat Support Care.* 2009;7(2):139–141.
23. Underwood LG, Teresi JA. The daily spiritual experience scale. *Annals Beh Med.* 2002;24:22–33.
24. Baider L, Holland JC, Russak SM, Kaplan De-Nour, A. The system of belief inventory (SBI-15). *Psycho-Oncol.* 2001;10:534–540.
25. McCullough ME, Larson DB. Religion and depression: a review of the literature. *Twin Res.* 1999;2:126–136.
26. Baider L, Russak SM, Perry S, et al. The role of religious and spiritual beliefs in coping with malignant melanoma: an Israeli sample. *Psychooncology* 1999;8:27–35.

27. Koenig HG, Cohen HJ, Blazer DG, et al. Religious coping and depression among elderly, hospitalized medically ill men. *Am J Psychiatry* 1992;149:1693–1700.

28. Koenig HG, George LK, Peterson BL. Religiosity and remission of depression in medically ill older patients. *Am J Psychiatry* 1998;155:536–542.

29. Baider L, Russak SM, Perry S et al. The role of religious and spiritual beliefs in coping with malignant melanoma: an Israeli sample. *Psychooncology,* 1999;8:27–35.

30. Chochinov HMC, et al. The landscape of distress in the terminally ill. *J Palliative Care Sympt Manage.* 2009;38(5):641–645.

31. Breitbart W, Rosenfeld B, Pessin H, et al. Depression, hopelessness, and desire for death in terminally ill patients with cancer. *JAMA* 2000;284:2907–2911.

32. McClain CS, Rosenfeld B, Breitbart W. Effect of spiritual well-being on end-of-life despair in terminally-ill cancer patients. *Lancet* 2003;361:1603–1607.

33. Balboni TA, Balboni M, Enzinger AC, et al. Provision of spiritual support to patients with advanced cancer by religious communities and associations with medical care at the end of life. *JAMA.* 2013;173(12):1109–1117.

34. Watson M, Haviland JJ, Greer S, et al. Influence of psychological response on survival in breast cancer population-based cohort study. *Lancet* 1999;354:1331–1336.

35. Chochinov HM, Wilson KG, Enns M, et al. Prevalence of depression in the terminally ill: effects of diagnostic criteria and symptom threshold judgments. *Am J Psychiatry* 1994;151:537–540.

36. Chochinov HM, Wilson KG, Enns M, et al. Desire for death in the terminally ill. *Am J Psychiatry* 1995;152:1185–1191.

37. Chochinov H, Wilson K, Enns M, et al. Depression, hopelessness, and suicidal ideation in the terminally ill. *Psychosomatics* 1998;39:366–370.

38. Rousseau P. Spirituality and the dying patient. *J Clin Oncol.* 2000;18:2000–2002.

39. Thiel MM, Robinson MR. Physicians' collaboration with chaplains: difficulties and benefits. *J Clin Ethics* 1997;8:94–103.

40. Yalom I. *Existential Psychotherapy.* New York: Basic Books; 1980.

41. Kissane DW, Poppito S. Death and dying. In: Blumenfield M, Strain JJ, eds. *Psychosomatic Medicine.* Philadelphia: Lippincott Williams & Wilkins; 2006:671–694.

42. Cherny NI. The treatment of suffering in patients with advanced cancer. In: Chochinov HMC, Breitbart W, eds. *Handbook of Psychiatry in Palliative Medicine,* 2nd ed. New York: Oxford University Press, 2009:300–323.

43. Kissane D, et al. Dignity, meaning and demoralization: Emerging paradigms in end of life care. In: Chochinov HMC, Breitbart W, eds. *Handbook of Psychiatry in Palliative Medicine,* 2nd ed. New York: Oxford University Press, 2009:324–340.

44. Breitbart W, Appelbaum A. Cancer care, meaning-centered group psychotherapy. In: Watson M, Kissane D, eds. *Handbook of Psychotherapy.* New York: Wiley-Blackwell; 2011:137–148.

Chapter 12

Cross-Cultural Issues

The term "culture" generally refers to the values, norms, habits, beliefs, and institutions that flow from a specific worldview and through which patterns of meaning are created.[1] Cultural heritage, religious beliefs, and social norms shape attitudes toward health, illness, and death. It is important to note that cultural background cannot solely predict any individual's experiences, beliefs, or attitudes. Culture is only a part of a complex series of factors, including gender, religion, life experiences, socioeconomic status, and individual psychology, all of which influence the way patients and health care professionals understand the experience of illness.[1] Culture provides a framework of expectations, including communication with health care providers, the decision-making process, and the illness itself.

Incorporating Cultural Differences into Palliative Care

Across cultures, the universal fear of cancer and other terminal illnesses is caused by the fear of death as well as images associated with debility and pain.[2] Yet individual societies place different emphases on issues surrounding death and dying. This cultural diversity has profound effects on decision-making processes at the end of life (Box 12.1).[3]

Individual as well as communal approaches to suffering and death are derived from culturally specific community systems and rituals.[6] For example, traditional Western cultures use coping strategies that are different from those of non-Western cultures.[7] These differences reflect varying degrees of emphasis on reliance on family and friends for social support, value of individual versus group effort, and the influence of spiritual and religious beliefs.[8]

Physicians from different geographical areas and diverse cultural backgrounds also hold culturally specific views on death and dying. A study comparing attitudes and beliefs of palliative care physicians from South America, Europe, and Canada suggests that there are major regional differences in the attitudes and beliefs of physicians regarding communication at the end of life.[5] This study revealed differences in attitudes toward truth telling, do not resuscitate orders, patients' willingness to know their diagnosis, and decision making at the end of life (Box 12.2).

In order to provide proper physical and emotional relief, psycho-oncologists must incorporate the patient's cultural beliefs into the evaluation and intervention process. It is the professional responsibility and ethical duty of the palliative care team to understand, respect, and honor the diversity of patients and their families.

The ABCDE model provides a framework and effective template for clinicians to incorporate cultural issues into the evaluation and treatment of patients (Box 12.3).[9]

Box 12.1 Culturally Specific Issues Surrounding Death and Dying

- Perception and interpretation of symptoms, treatment, pain, and suffering[4]
- Patient's willingness to know diagnosis and prognosis
- Doctor's willingness to discuss diagnosis and prognosis
- Decision-making roles among health care team, patient, and family[4]
- Communication among physician, patient, and family[5]
- Spiritual and religious rituals and traditions
- Grief and bereavement

Box 12.2 European, South American, and Canadian Palliative Care Physicians' Attitudes Regarding End-of-Life Care[5]

- Although all three groups of physicians agreed all cancer patients should be informed of their diagnosis, European and South American physicians reported that not all of their patients knew their diagnosis.
- Although all three groups believed "do not resuscitate" orders should be discussed with the patient in all cases, European physicians were least likely to obtain a "do not resuscitate" order regarding their patients.
- Although all three groups of physicians agreed that a joint decision-making strategy was most appropriate, South American physicians reported less joint decision making than Canadian and European physicians.
- European and South American physicians strongly disagreed with Canadian physicians in the belief that:
  - Terminally ill patients want to be informed of the true nature of their illness.
  - Families are willing to inform the patient of the terminal nature of illness.

Box 12.3 Evaluation of Cultural Issues: ABCDE Model[9]

Attitudes

Elicit *a*ttitudes about illness, family care, and responsibilities.

Beliefs

Explore *b*eliefs and ritual practices.

Ask direct questions about faith and religious experience; follow up on cues.

Do not respond to statements of religious and spiritual values with facts. Reflect them respectfully.

Do not deny or pretend to go along with expectations such as miracles, but use statements that indicate a shared desire for the best outcome that can be arranged.

Context

Inquire about the cultural *c*ontext in which the patient and family operate.

Decisions

Determine the patient's *d*ecision-making style.

Environment

Learn about the patient's current environment.

Delivering Culturally Sensitive Palliative Care around the World

There is a growing need for developing culturally sensitive palliative care services. Cultural and ethnic disparities in cancer care, management of pain and other symptoms, and hospice utilization have been well documented in the literature.[1] Developing culturally sensitive palliative care services is a giant step toward eliminating the disparities across different cultures. Several countries across the globe have started working toward that goal. This is exemplified in the translation of quality-of-life measures into languages other than English.[6] Furthermore, palliative care teams have integrated cultural traditions for treating spiritual, existential, and physical pain into modern techniques for relieving pain and suffering. Psycho-oncologists must be aware of the diversity of cultural beliefs that greatly influence the experience of death and dying among various populations.

The following sections introduce several cultural issues that psycho-oncologists should be aware of when interacting with patients of different cultural backgrounds. However, there remains a great need for culturally sensitive end-of-life care research that may help improve palliative care around the world.

North America

United States

There are more than 4,000 hospices, more than 1,000 hospital-based pain and palliative care services, and several other palliative care delivery systems that serve more than a million patients in the United States. The diversity of the patient population presents cultural issues and barriers that health care providers must face when providing palliative care (Box 12.4).

Because of the cultural diversity within the United States, studies have explored cultural views of death and dying. North American patients are generally told the diagnosis of cancer and the most accurate prognosis known by their physician.[5] However, even within the United States, different ethnic groups have varying opinions of how appropriate it is for physicians to share the terminal diagnosis with patients and families. This directly influences how palliative care teams can provide culturally sensitive care. The Witness Project cancer education program for African-American women is a prime example of a culturally sensitive approach to medical care.[13] This culturally competent cancer education program partners with local church leaders to educate African-American women about cancer screening, treatments, and palliative care.

African Americans

The African-American population in the United States is known to face greater discrimination and more barriers than other ethnic groups within the US health care system. Studies suggest that they have a low level of trust of the health care system because of personal experience with poor access to medical care and awareness of abuses in medical research in the past, such as the

Box 12.4 Issues in Palliative Care That Are Influenced by Cultural Factors in the United States

- Role of patient in decision making:[10–19]
  - Patient autonomy
  - Informed consent
- Role of family in decision making
  - Nondisclosure about cancer illness
- Physician-patient relationship
  - Role of physician in decision making
  - Communication between the physician and patient/family
  - Patient mistrust of physicians
- Expression of pain
- Attitudes toward suffering
- Spiritual and religious traditions
- Appropriateness of openly naming disease or discussing death

Tuskegee syphilis study.[10] This mistrust may influence decisions for end-of-life care. Specifically, African Americans may be less likely to complete advance directives than white respondents because of a negative view of advance directives.[11,20–24] They also have a stronger preference for the use of life support than other racial groups.[1,25–27] African Americans have been shown to utilize hospice services less frequently compared with white patients.[28] African Americans, compared with Korean Americans and Mexican Americans, favor a patient autonomy model.[12] They are more likely to believe a patient should be told the diagnosis of metastatic cancer and that a patient should be told of a terminal prognosis.

Studies also suggest that African Americans use different coping mechanisms when facing a terminal illness. African Americans often turn to God and the church for support and assistance when facing life-threatening illnesses. African Americans with chronic pain use hope and pray more than whites with chronic pain.[13] In a study on religious activity and depression among elderly African Americans and whites with serious physical illness, results suggest attending religious services had a greater impact on the positive affect and depression among African Americans compared with whites.

Hispanics

Like African Americans, Hispanics also have different coping mechanisms when faced with a terminal illness. Puerto Rican cancer patients were found to cope differently than whites.[14] Hispanics are more likely to rely on religion as a means of coping. Many Hispanics express spirituality through organized religion, particularly Roman Catholicism. However, Hispanics also often utilize folk healers, such as *Curanderas* (Mexican Americans), *Spiritualists* (Puerto Ricans), and *Santeras* (Cuban Americans). These healers represent a belief system with roots in American-Indian, African, and Catholic faiths and should be viewed as important components of overall treatment for patients who utilize them.[15]

Hispanics also have culturally specific views of death and dying. Hispanics are less likely to express comfort in discussing end-of-life issues with their physicians than white or African-American patients.[16] Not only do Hispanics support the view that doctors should not discuss death and dying, but they rely on a family-centered model of medical decision making.[12] The family's role is meant to remove the burden of making treatment decisions from patient, which may involve keeping information about the disease and prognosis from the patient.[11] In a study of Mexican-American patients and families, the families felt it was their duty to protect the patient and make the patient comfortable and free of distress at the end of life.[17]

Hispanics tend to have DNR orders and advance directives less frequently than non-Hispanic white patients.[29] Hispanics have been found to be less likely to favor withdrawal of life support when compared with white patients.[30] Hispanics are less likely to use hospice services compared with non-Hispanic white patients.[31]

Asian Americans

Similar to Hispanics, Asian Americans also hold a family-centered model of medical decision making and often do not think it is appropriate for doctors to discuss issues of death and dying with the patient.[12] Chinese-American families often feel that it is their duty to protect the patient and prevent any distress at the end of life.[17] Therefore, disclosure of prognosis and diagnosis are often discouraged.[11] However, this effect decreases with acculturation, as is seen with Japanese Americans, who were also found to have positive attitudes toward advance care planning.[18]

Korean Americans have been found to be less likely to favor withdrawal or withholding of life support.[30] Asian Americans are less likely to utilize hospice services compared with white patients.

Native Americans

Native Americans perceive disclosure of terminal illness to be negative.[19] Therefore, communication between the doctor and patient is often discouraged if there is an unfavorable diagnosis. This cultural view is reflected in studies that show that Native Americans rejected advance directives because care planning would be a violation of cultural values of avoidance of negative thinking and speaking.[19]

The differences in advance care directives, willingness to withdraw or withhold life support, and hospice utilization among African-American, Asian-American, and Hispanic-American minorities have been attributed to a variety of factors, including the lack of knowledge on end-of-life issues, low socioeconomic status, patients' and families' attitudes toward terminal illness, and unavailability of bilingual staff on-site.[1] The underlying reasons for disparities in provision of palliative care among minorities are clearly complex. However, the finding that palliative care services have steadily improved in the last two decades among minority groups is encouraging and calls for further studies in this area.[32]

Canada

In Canada, there is much support for a high level of information for patients regarding diagnosis and prognosis.[5] In a study of views of sedation at the end of life, Canadian physicians, patients, and families valued clearer thinking and full disclosure of information.[33] Most palliative care physicians thus work in an environment in which most patients are aware of their diagnosis of cancer. These studies also suggest that patient autonomy is an important ethical decision-making principle within matters of end-of-life care.[5]

South America

The cultural values of Latin American countries focus on interdependence, collectivism, and nondisclosure rather than on a patient's independent judgment, autonomy, and full disclosure. There is a paternalistic pattern of practicing medical decision making as well as an increased concern about financial status and access to health care.[34]

In the Latin American culture, there is a complex relationship between health and illness, death and dying, as well as the physical, mental, and spiritual aspects of an individual's life embedded in a particular system of belief (Box 12.5).[35]

Peru

The Matsigenka, a mountain people on the eastern slopes of the Peruvian Andes, hold unique beliefs about death and dying. There is great anxiety over the contagion of death and the power of the dead over the living. The Matsigenka believe that ghosts temporarily roam the liminal space between life and death. Excessive displays of emotion, especially grief, anger, and aggressive sexuality, cause a vicious cycle of unhappiness, social disruption, illness, and death.[37]

Argentina

There is an increasing need for palliative care in Argentina, especially because two out of three deaths are caused by chronic diseases, including different types of cancer.[38] Although the health system in Argentina is complex and evolving, there is a lack of palliative care programs that help patient-family units with physical, social, and emotional needs at the end of life.[39]

Obstacles to providing palliative care include patients and families receiving inadequate information about their diagnosis or prognosis.[38] This may be influenced by a culturally specific view regarding communication among physicians, patients, and patient families. In a study comparing attitudes of communication among physicians from Argentina, Europe, and Canada, Argentinian physicians favored patient-based decision making less frequently when compared with Canadian physicians.[5] These physicians reported more decision making by doctors. Although these physicians believed that patients should be aware of both diagnosis and terminal stage of illness, they reported that patients did not know about the terminal nature of their illness.

Europe

Issues surrounding care for dying patients in Europe are similar to those of patients in North America. A recent review of cultural and regional variations

Box 12.5 Cultural Views Relevant to Palliative Care in Latin America[36]

- Family involvement is basic and vital. The family-centered model of decision making is fundamental and more important and relevant than patient autonomy. This is called *fatalismo*, which is characterized by interdependency, affiliation, and cooperation.
- Extended family members and relatives actively participate in the spiritual and physical care of an ill family member.
- The family often hears the medical news before the patient is informed so that they can gradually shield the patient from the "bad" news.
- The family and patient will be at home at the end of life. There is a cultural belief that the hospital setting is impersonal and disrupts the family's ability to take care of their loved one.
- Families and patients often believe that God determines the outcome of illness and death as a natural part of the life process. This belief also serves as a protective role by preparing the patient and family for grief and death.
- Respect (*respeto*) is a very important concept in the Latin culture and throughout the care and death process.

associated with end-of-life issues found that although recent European laws have emphasized patient autonomy, advance care planning is rarely used.[28] Decisions are often made by physicians, nurses, and families. This study proposed a European "north-to-south" gradient in paternalism in the decision-making process and emphasized the influence of religious beliefs on end-of-life decisions. This supports the large variation in the extent to which end-of-life decisions are discussed with patients, relatives, and other caregivers throughout European countries such as Belgium, Denmark, Italy, the Netherlands, Sweden, and Switzerland.[40]

The United Kingdom

A study assessing palliative care needs and perspectives of patients, informal care providers, and health care providers found that there were difficulties in communication and information exchange.[41] Informal caregivers were also less likely to receive full information about the illness and its progression, suggesting a patient-centered decision-making model.

France

Recent legislation passed in 2005 supports the trend in Europe toward patient autonomy and full disclosure of information before treatment.[42] This law not only reinforces the role of both the patient's surrogate decision maker, but also emphasizes that the patient's advance directive establishes consent.

Spain

Studies of Spain and other countries with a Latin cultural background have observed that the role played by families of terminal patients and the attitude toward information and diagnosis disclosure is different from the Northern

European or North American model.[43] Researchers argue that although religion may no longer play a predominant source of these cultural differences, these differences may be caused by remaining Catholic influences ingrained in the culture. For example, the term "hospice" may have negative connotations because the term denotes either extreme poverty or orphanage.

Cultural factors influence issues surrounding end-of-life care, such as the widespread acceptance of pain relief to the point of sedation. In a study on sedation at the end of life, there were major differences between Spanish and Canadian patients.[33] Spanish patients sought sedation for psychological and existential distress. This may be caused by differences in views of disclosure of information and cognition between patients and families.

Italy

Many studies have been done to explore the attitudes and practices of Italian patients and physicians toward information and communication. Until 1990, it was common practice in Italy to withhold truth from cancer patients in order to protect them and maintain their hope.[44–46] Within such a community-centered culture, individual autonomy was perceived as isolation.[44] However, Italian culture has substantially evolved toward a patient-centered model: patients expect and receive more complete information and are more involved in their own medical care.[47]

Asia and Pacific

Palliative care programs and services are expanding in Asia. These services are often influenced by cultural views that favor a family-centered model of care.

China

Considering the family as the unit of care, rather than the individual, is of paramount importance in Chinese society. Patients within the family keep their psychological and emotional problems of illness and death to themselves. This is related to their desire to avoid upsetting others and so promoting harmony in a stressful situation. The Chinese believe that emotions must be contained and controlled.[48]

For hundreds of years in China, ancestral rituals at the family altar and grave were the means by which the dead interceded with higher powers on behalf of the living. Cultural dimensions of death, dying, and bereavement included the following themes: (1) saving face (the more restraint shown in mourning for the deceased, the more the person was loved); (2) filial piety (duty to one's relative); and (3) invoking luck, blessing, and fortune (belief in life, afterlife, and the presence of spirit).[49]

Japan

Barriers to the provision of palliative and hospice care exist at both the individual and organization levels in terms of reimbursement incentives from the national insurance system. In a survey of physicians they described the feeling of being unprepared to deal with the emotional needs of patients and families, having to make medical decisions, facing time pressures, fear of making a mistake, and a sense of failure related to patients' lack of improvement.[50]

Korea

In a study on attitudes of cancer patients and their families toward disclosure of terminal illness to the patient, cancer patients want to be informed if their illness is terminal.[51] They often want to be informed immediately after the diagnosis. Palliative care physicians should be aware that there might be differences in the patient and family attitude toward disclosure.

Nepal

In Nepal, the traditional view of disclosure suggests that physicians do not discuss diagnoses of malignancy with their patients.[52] Physicians should discuss the diagnosis with family members, who filter the information and communicate the news to the patient. This may result in a disparity between what patients would like to be told if they should develop cancer and what patients actually know about their diagnosis.

India

Traditional palliative care in India, practiced in the home, includes spiritual and religious care according to traditional customs and rituals.[53] These traditional views often discourage the use of opiates, which poses a challenge for providing pain relief and symptom control in cancer patients.[54] Palliative care also involves the family in medical decision making. Thus, patient preferences and decisions are often influenced by family members at the end of life.[53]

Australia

With more than 500 language groups in existence before European settlement in the late 1700s, Australia is a culturally diverse country that is encouraging cultural competency in health. In a national guide to promote cultural competency, attention was given to particular populations within Australia.[55] For example, studies on migrants have identified psychosocial risk factors associated with stresses of settlement. These psychosocial risk factors include alienation, isolation, lack of social and family support networks, change of traditional roles within the family, and communication difficulties.

Much attention has also been given to the relatively poor health outcomes and unique needs of Aboriginal and Torres Strait Islanders. The Aboriginal and Torres Strait Islander peoples view culture as a central element in their perceptions of health and ill health. Their views of death and dying greatly differ from those of the dominant Anglo-Australian population.[56] For example, Aborigines often invoke sorcery and search for the "meaning, not mechanisms" of illness.[57]

Specific cultural factors pose challenges to delivering palliative care to Aboriginal communities. In Aboriginal communities, blame for a death or the attribution of cause of death affects decision making and conflict resolution at the end of life.[56] Palliative care workers are often reluctant to deliver care to patients because of the fear of blame. With regard to grief and bereavement, death is so frequent that some Aboriginal communities are in either acute or chronic shock from constant bereavement.[57] Because of the close community ties, every death inflicts a considerable degree of grief and sadness on large numbers of people. These cultural factors must be considered when providing palliative care at the end of life.

Middle East

Muslim Arab families are directly involved in caring for loved ones who are facing illness and impending death. Being a burden to the family is not the family's or the patient's concern. Thus when confronted with cancer illness, most Muslim Arabs will not go to nursing homes or hospices.[58] Instead, they remain at home and are tended by females who are expected to provide all the care.

End-of-life care is not only influenced by strong family ethics, but also by Islamic ethics. These ethical principles are intimately linked to the broad religious teachings of the Qur'an and the tradition of the Prophet Muhammad. These principles are inseparable from the religion and are based on duties and obligations to God and family as an expected and irrefutable law (Box 12.6).

Saudia Arabia

In Saudi Arabia, religious care is an integral part of palliative care and plays a valuable role in helping the patient cope with terminal illness. The support from the family enhances the patient's ability to cope with the disease and gives a higher level of life satisfaction. The most pervasive influence on health care provided in an Islamic community is Islam.

The family constitutes the dominant social institution through which persons inherit their religious, class, and cultural affiliations. The very concept of family in the Arab Muslim world reflects mutual commitments and relationships of interdependency and reciprocity.[60]

Pakistan

In Pakistani Muslim society, it is normal and expected that the family rather than the patient take center stage in the process of terminal illness. The physician—*shahib* (Lord)—shares the authority with the family as an equal partner in

Box 12.6 Cultural and Religious Values Influence Palliative Care in Muslims[58,59]

- Muslims have values based on the laws of the Qur'an.
- To maintain harmony is to accept hierarchical relations based on family kinship.
- Arab heritage is based on shared loyalty, unquestionable family authority by males, and kinship bonds.
- Friends and any social contacts are considered secondary to total commitment to family.
- It is normative behavior for the family to be responsible for the care of the patient.
- Being a burden to the family is not the family's or the patient's concern.
- It is expected that the females provide all the caregiving to the patient and male family members.
- When confronted with cancer illness, most Muslim Arabs will not go to nursing homes or hospices.

decision making. The family and the physician will generally protect the patient from anxiety and distress associated with the knowledge of impending death.[50]

The individual is viewed as sociocentrically enmeshed in inextricable social bonds, ties that make interpersonal process the source of vital decision in illness and death.[61]

Africa

Palliative care programs are continuing to be established in Africa. These programs often offer palliative care for individuals with AIDS and cancer. The unavailability of opioids and a lack of education of health care workers challenge the delivery of palliative care in Africa, especially in developing countries.[62,63] Nonetheless, many patients seem to value the support given by their families, communities, and religious fellowships.

Uganda

Home care programs and palliative care services have been established in Uganda to identify and meet the palliative care needs of the terminally ill. In a study focused in Kimpala, most of the participants had either HIV/AIDS or cancer or both. Patients identified that a "good death" involved when a dying person is being cared for at home, is free from pain and other distressing symptoms, is at peace, and has his or her basic needs met without feeling dependent on others.[64]

Kenya

The attitudes toward palliative care may differ greatly in developing countries such as Kenya. In a study comparing the experiences and needs of terminally ill patients in Scotland and Kenya, Kenyan patients were highly concerned about analgesia, essential equipment, suitable food, and assistance with care.[63] Kenyan patients felt that their social, spiritual, and psychological needs were met by families, local community, and religious groups. Dying patients in Eastern Kenya also reported that support structures helped them meet emotional, social, and spiritual needs at the end of life.[65] However, these patients described a "good death" as one that involves accessible pain relief, affordable clinic or inpatient care, and help to cope with the burden of care.

Summary

Fundamental values and beliefs vary across cultures. People are conscious of certain explicit beliefs, values, and associated behaviors. Other beliefs, values, and associated behaviors function at a more routine and grounded level of implicit norms. Culture hides much more than it reveals, and strangely enough what it hides, it hides most effectively from its own participants. Only when encountering another person or group with a different operating system does one realize the difference. The other person does not behave or speak the same.

When it comes to medical care, patients belonging to a particular cultural group may sense that the health team is acting with an unfamiliar set of norms, whereas the health team professionals most likely are unaware of their "peculiar" behavior. Negotiating a mutually acceptable approach to care can be particularly challenging, because participants perceive another reality and frequently do not realize the position from which they are negotiating.[66,67] Promoting cultural awareness and cultural competence among health care professionals should improve their confidence and skills in providing comprehensive care for patients and families from different backgrounds.[68] Cultural competence is effective when based on knowledge of a culture, appreciation of cultural differences, awareness of biases and prejudices, and attitudes of humility, empathy, curiosity, respect, and sensitivity.[69] It should be noted that the validity of a description of an encounter between individuals from diverse cultures may be weakened, because it may be based on relatively limited information filtered through one's own environmental predisposition.[69] Culturally unprepared outsiders might misinterpret extraordinarily traditional customs as being the social norm. They might also draw conclusions based on interpreting an event or pattern of behavior out of its cultural context. In turn, the insiders' views of their own culture are likely to be tinged with positively charged judgmental bias. This, however, does not negate the possibility that a culture could be described more accurately by integrating the view from within with an outside perspective.[69]

In adapting to change and adversity, societies draw on experiences and coping resources developed over the course of time, influenced by ethnicity and components of culture, group history, social status, group heritage, and systems of belief. When defined in this way, culture functions as an integrating force for individuals passing through significant life changes, providing a context for evaluating issues of health and illness, and death and dying.[70] It is crucial for health care providers to recognize the influence of cultural factors and be able to provide culturally sensitive palliative care.

References

1. Blackhall LJ. Cultural diversity and palliative care. In: Chochinov HMC, Breitbart W, eds. *Handbook of Psychiatry in Palliative Medicine*, 2nd ed. New York: Oxford University Press; 2009:186–201.
2. Butow P, Tattersall M, Goldstein D. Communication with cancer patients in culturally diverse societies. *Ann NY Acad Sci*. 1997;809:317–329.
3. Krakauer E, Crenner C, Fox K. Barriers to optimum end-of-life care for minority patients. *J Am Geriatric Soc*. 2002;50(1):182–190.
4. Marshall PA, Koenig BA, Barnes DM, Davis AJ. Multiculturalism, bioethics and end-of-life care: narratives of Latino cancer patients. In: Monagle JF, Thomasma DC, eds. *Health Care Ethics: Issues for the 21st Century*. Gaithersburg, MD: Aspen; 1998:421–431.
5. Bruera E, Neumann CM, Mazzocato C, Stiefel F, Sala R. Attitudes and beliefs of palliative care physicians regarding communication with terminally ill cancer patients. *Palliat Med*. 2000;14(4):287–298.
6. Stjernsward J, Clark D. Palliative medicine: a global perspective. In: Doyle D, Hanks G, Cherny N, Calman K, 3rd ed. *Oxford Textbook of Palliative Medicine*. New York: Oxford University Press; 2004:1199–1224.
7. Barg FK, Gullate MM. Cancer support groups: meeting the needs of African Americans with cancer. *Semin Oncol Nurs*. 2001;17(3):171–178.

8. Mazanec P, Tyler MK. Cultural considerations in end-of-life care. *Am J Nurs.* 2003;103(3):50–58.
9. Koenig BA, Gates-Williams J. Understanding cultural differences in caring for dying patients. *West J Med.* 1995;163(3):244–224.
10. Berger JT. Culture and ethnicity in clinical care. *Arch Intern Med.* 1998;158(19):2085–2090.
11. Kwak J, Haley WE. Current research findings on end-of-life decision making among racially or ethnically diverse groups. *Gerontologist* 2005;45(5):634–641.
12. Blackhall LJ, Murphy ST, Frank G, et al. Ethnicity and attitudes toward patient autonomy. *JAMA.* 1995;274;820–825.
13. Erwin DO. Cancer education takes on a spiritual focus for the African-American faith community. *J Cancer Educ.* 2002;17:46–49.
14. Ell KO, Nishimoto RH. Coping resources in adaptation to cancer: socio-economic and racial differences. *Soc Serv Rev.* 1989;63:433–446.
15. Canive JM, Castillo D. Hispanic veterans diagnosed with PTSD: assessment and treatment issues. *NCCP Clin Qrtly.* 1997;7, 1.
16. Morrison RS, Zayas LH, Mulyihill M, Baskin SA, Meier DE. Barriers to completion of health care proxies: an examination of ethnic differences. *Arch Intern Med.* 1998;158(22):2493–2497.
17. Orona CJ, Koenig BA, Davis AJ. Cultural aspects of nondisclosure. *Cambridge Qrtly Healthcare Ethics.* 1994;3:338–346.
18. Matsumura S, Bito S, Liu H, et al. Acculturation of attitudes toward end-of-life care: a cross-cultural survey of Japanese Americans and Japanese. *J Gen Intern Med.* 2002;17(7):531–539.
19. Carrese JA, Rhodes LA. Western bioethics on the Navajo reservation. Benefit or harm? *JAMA.* 1995;274(10):826–829.
20. Wenger NS, Pearson ML, et al. Epidemiology of do not resuscitate orders: disparity by age, diagnosis, gender, race, and functional impairment. *Arch Intern Med* 1995;155:2056–2062.
21. Phillips RS, Teno J, Oye RK. Choices of seriously ill patients about cardiopulmonary resuscitation: correlates and outcomes. *Am J Med* 1996;100:128–137.
22. Rosenfeld KE, Wenger NS, Phillips RS, et al. Factors associated with change in resuscitation preference of seriously ill patients. *Arch Intern Med* 1996;156:1558–1564.
23. Wenger NS, Oye RK, Desbiens RS, et al. The stability of DNR orders on hospital readmission. *J Clin Ethics* 1996;7:48–54.
24. Zingmond DS, Wenger NS. Regional and institutional variation in the initiation of early do not resuscitate orders. *Arch Intern Med* 2005;165:1705–1712.
25. Goodlin SJ, Zhong Z, et al. Factors associated with use of cardiopulmonary resuscitation in seriously ill hospitalized adults. *JAMA.* 1999;282:2333–2339.
26. Gessert CE, Curry NM, Robinson A. Ethnicity and end of life care: the use of feeding tubes. *Ethn Dis.* 2001;11:97–106.
27. Phipps E, True G, Harris D, et al. Approaching the end of life: attitudes, preferences, and behaviors of African-American and white patients and their family caregivers. *J Clin Oncol.* 2003;21:549–551.
28. Virnig BA, Morgan RO, Persily NA, et al. Racial and income differences in the use of the hospice benefit between the Medicare managed care and Medicare fee-for-service. *J Palliat Med.* 1999;2:23–31.

29. Kiely DK, Mitchell CL, Marlow A, et al. Racial and state differences in the designation of advance directives in nursing home residents. *J Am Geriatr Soc.* 2001;49:1346–1352.

30. Blackhall L, Frank G, Palmer J, et al. Ethnicity and attitudes towards withholding and withdrawing medical care. *Soc Sci Med.* 1999;48(12):1979–1989.

31. Haas JS, Earle CC, Orav JE. Lower use of hospice by cancer patients who live in minority versus white areas. *J Gen Intern Med.* 2007;22:396–399.

32. Lackan NA, Ostir GV, Freeman JL, et al. Decreasing variation in the use of hospice among older adults with breast, colorectal, lung, and prostate cancer. *Med Care* 2004;42:116–122.

33. Fainsinger RL, Nú ñez-Olarte JM, Demoissac DM. The cultural differences in perceived value of disclosure and cognition: Spain and Canada. *J Palliat Care* 2003;19(1):43–48.

34. Wenk R, Bertolino M. Argentina: palliative care status 2002. *J Pain Symptom Manage.* 2002;24:166–169.

35. Lobar SL, Youngblut JM, Brooten D. Cross-cultural beliefs, ceremonies and rituals surrounding death of a loved one. *Pediatric Nurs* 2006;32(1):44–50.

36. Vasquez MA, Williams PJ. The power of religious identities in the Americas. *Latin Amer Perspect.* 2005;32(1):5–26.

37. Shepard GH Jr. Three days for weeping: dreams, emotions, and death in the Peruvian Amazon. *Med Anthrop Qrtly.* 2002;16(2):200–229.

38. De Simone GG. Palliative care in Argentina: perspectives from a country in crisis. *J Pain Palliat Care Pharmacother.* 2003;17(3–4):23–43.

39. Wenk R, Bertolino M. Palliative care development in South America: a focus on Argentina. *J Pain Symptom Manage.* 2007;33(5):645–50.

40. Van der Heide A, Deliens L, Faisst K. End-of-life decision-making in six European countries: descriptive study. *Lancet* 2003;362:345–350.

41. McIlfatrick S. Assessing palliative care needs: views of patients, informal carers and healthcare professionals. *J Adv Nurs.* 2007;57(1):77–86.

42. Franchitto N, Vinour H, Gavarri L, Telmon N, Rouge D. End-of-life patients, intensive care and consent: difficulties facing French intensivists. *Eur J Anaesthesiol.* 2007;24(8):709–713.

43. Núñez Olarte JM, Guillen DG. Cultural issues and ethical dilemmas in palliative and end-of-life care in Spain. *Cancer Control* 2001;81:46–54.

44. Surbone A. Truth telling to the patient. *JAMA.* 1992;268:1661–1662.

45. Surbone A. The information to the cancer patient: psychosocial and spiritual implications. *Support Care Cancer* 1993;1:89–91.

46. Gordon DR, Paci E. Disclosure practice and cultural narratives: understanding concealment and silence around cancer in Tuscany, Italy. *Soc Sci Med.* 1997;44:1433–1452.

47. Mosconi P, Meyerowitz BE, Liberati MC, et al. Disclosure of breast cancer diagnosis: patient and physician reports. *Ann Oncol.* 1991;2:273–280.

48. Liu J-E, Mok E, Wong T. Perceptions of supportive communication in Chinese patients with cancer: experiences and expectations. *J Adv Nurs.* 2005;52(3):262–270.

49. Klass D, Goss R. The Politics of grief and continuing bonds with the dead: the cases of Maoist China and Wahhabi Islam. *Death Studies* 2003;27:787–811.

50. Schreiner AS, Hara N, Terakado T, Ikegami N. Attitudes towards end-of-life care in a geriatric hospital in Japan. *Int J Palliat Nurs.* 2004;10(4):185–193.

51. Yun YH, Lee CG, Kim SY, et al. The attitudes of cancer patients and their families toward the disclosure of terminal illness. *J Clin Oncol.* 2004;22(2):307–314.
52. Gongal R, Vaidya P, Jha R, Rajbhandary O, Watson M. Informing patients about cancer in Nepal: what do people prefer? *Palliat Med.* 2006;20(4):471–476.
53. Chaturvedi SK, Chandra PS. Palliative care in India. *Support Care Cancer.* 1998;6(2):81–84.
54. Joransen DE, Gilson AM, Maurer MA. Improving opioid availability. *Ind J Palliat Care* 2005;11:119–120.
55. Australian Government National Health and Medical Research Council. *Cultural Competency in Health: A Guide for Policy, Partnerships, and Participation.* Canberra, ACT: Commonwealth of Australia; 2006.
56. McGrath CL. Issues influencing the provision of palliative care services to remote aboriginal communities in the Northern Territory. *Aust J Rural Hlth.* 2002;8(1):24–51.
57. Weeramanthri T. Practice guidelines for health professionals dealing with the death of a Northern Territory Aboriginal Person. *Menzies Occasional Papers.* Northern Territory: Menzies School of Health Research; 1996:1, 96.
58. Duffy SA, Jackson FC, Schim SM, Ronis DL, Fowler KE. Racial/ethnic preferences, sex preferences, and perceived discrimination related to end-of-life care. *J Am Geriatr Soc.* 2006;54(1):150–157.
59. Nydell MK. *Understanding Arabs*, 3rd ed. Yarmouth, ME: Intercultural Press; 2002.
60. Al-Shahri M. The future of palliative care in the Islamic world. *West J Med.* 2002;176(1):60–61.
61. Al-Shahri MZ, Al-Khenaizan A. Palliative care for Muslim patients. *J Support Oncol.* 2005;3(6):432–436.
62. Livingstone H. Pain relief in the developing world: the experience of hospice Africa-Uganda. *J Pain Palliat Care Pharmacother.* 2003;17(3–4):107–118.
63. Murray SA, Grant E, Grant A, Kendall M. Dying from cancer in developed and developing countries: lessons from two qualitative interview studies of patients and their careers. *BMJ.* 2003;326(7385):368.
64. Kikule E. A good death in Uganda: survey of needs for palliative care in urban areas. *BMJ.* 2003;327:192–194.
65. Grant E, Murray SA, Grant A, Brown J. A good death in rural Kenya? Listening to Meru patients and their families talk about care needs at the end of life. *J Palliat Care.* 2003;19(3):159–167.
66. Hallenbeck JL. Intercultural differences and communication at the end of life. *Prim Care* 2001;2(28):401–413.
67. Kagawa-Singer M, Blackhall LJ. Negotiating cross-cultural issues at the end of life. *JAMA.* 2001;286:2993–3001.
68. Surbone A. Cultural competence: why? *Ann Oncol.* 2004;15:697–699.
69. Surbone A. Cultural aspects of communication in cancer care. In Stiefel F, ed. *Recent Results in Cancer Research.* Heidelberg: Springer-Verlag; 2006:91–104.
70. Triandis HC. *Culture and Social Behavior.* New York: McGraw-Hill; 1994.

Chapter 13

Doctor-Patient Communication in Palliative Care

Doctor-patient communication is an essential component in caring for a dying patient.[1–7] Several studies have focused on doctor-patient communication during the dying process. In the absence of good communication, patients and families cannot make informed decisions.

Poor communication between cancer patients and their physicians may cause cancer patients to overestimate their prognosis and misinterpret treatment choices (Box 13.1).[8]

Communication problems have been identified in 84% to 94% of clinical encounters. Patients with cancer and their families have reported *unmet communication needs* for information about the extent of disease, prognosis, treatment options, intent, and adverse effects.[9,10]

Despite the recognized importance of caregiver-patient communication, many physicians are not adequately trained in communication. In a study of oncologists' communication skills, less than 35% of oncologists reported having received any previous communication training.[7] However, this study did find that most oncologists desire to learn better communication techniques and are willing to sacrifice the necessary time to do so.

Good doctor-patient communication reduces risk of iatrogenic suffering, mood, anxiety, and adjustment disorders among cancer patients and their families (Boxes 13.2–13.4).[1,11,12]

Buckman emphasizes the importance of teaching and practicing listening skills, using comforting body language, responding empathically to patients, and engaging in therapeutic and supportive dialogue (Boxes 13.5–13.7).[3]

Most recently, several intensive training programs in doctor-patient communication have been demonstrated to have both short- and long-term efficacy in improving communication skills among physicians and other health care professionals (Boxes 13.8 and 13.9).[9,17–19]

The communication skills training program at Memorial Sloan Kettering Cancer Center is a structured communications initiative that is designed to find the most effective and lasting way to train health care professionals to communicate in a sensitive and productive manner. A dedicated staff of facilitators as well as dedicated laboratory space, which includes a classroom and six

Box 13.1 Patients' Predictions of Prognosis Influence Treatment Decisions[8]

- Patients with terminal lung and colon cancer overestimated their probability of surviving 6 months, and these overestimations influenced their treatment decisions.
- Patients who believed that they were going to live more than 6 months were more likely to choose aggressive, life-extending therapy than were patients who believed that they had less than a 10% chance of living beyond 6 months. The latter patients were more likely to choose comfort care.
- The survival rate for those who opted for aggressive treatment was lower than the survival rate for those who chose comfort care.

Box 13.2 Benefits of Improved Doctor-Patient Communication

- Improved training in doctor-patient communication can help ease anxiety on both sides and improve health outcomes.[13]
- Improving physicians' empathic responses to patients in medical interviews can improve the doctor-patient relationship, improve quality of care, and increase both physician and patient satisfaction.[14]

Box 13.3 Specific Doctor-Patient Communication Problems

Problems in identifying patient concerns[1,9,10,15]

Problems with delivering information (discrepancy among the patient's actual need, concerns for information and the doctor's assumption of the patient's need for information, and the patient's concerns regarding the information delivered)[1,15,16]

video-recording training rooms, strives to provide communication skills training to health care professionals (Box 13.10).

Breaking bad news is one of the most difficult and challenging communication tasks that clinicians struggle with on a daily basis. Many clinicians find the Six-Step Protocol for Breaking Bad News extremely useful (Box 13.11). This protocol can be used by psycho-oncologists when they teach communication skills to physicians in the palliative care setting.

Box 13.4 Guidelines for Communication and Empathy in Caring for the Dying Patient[1,3,4]

1. *Important elements of communication in palliative care:*
   Basic listening skills
   Breaking bad news
   Therapeutic dialogue
   Communicating with the family and with other professionals
2. *Sources of difficulty when communicating with a dying patient:*
   Social denial of death
   Lack of experience of death in the family
   High expectations of health and life
   Materialism
   The changing role of religion
   The patient's fear of dying
   The patient's and the family's unfamiliarity with medical knowledge
3. *Factors originating in the health care professional:*[1,9,16–18]
   Failure to establish trust
   Failure to establish patient/family's perspective
   Clinician avoidance/switching the topic
   Normalization/premature reassurance
   Sympathetic pain
   Fear of being blamed
   Fear of the untaught or lack of training
   Fear of expressing emotions
   Fear of harming the patient
   Fear of one's own illness and death
   Lack of emotional support

Box 13.5 Definition of Basic Empathic Skills Necessary for Meaningful Communication with Patients[14]

"...recognizing when emotions may be present but not directly expressed, inviting exploration of these unexpressed feelings, and effectively acknowledging these feelings so that the patient feels understood."

Box 13.6 Key Strategies for Effective Doctor-Patient Communication[1]

- Developing and sustaining trust through preserving dignity of the patient and family and eliciting and treating suffering
- Giving the patient and family choice whether/when/how much to discuss sensitive issues
- Treating the patient and family with the utmost respect
- Checking the patient's awareness of the diagnosis, prognosis, and treatment options
- Eliciting the patient's concerns and feelings

Box 13.7 Core Communication Skills[9]

- Agenda setting: Declare and invite agenda items.
- Check for understanding and preference for information (readiness to discuss management options). ASK-TELL-ASK
- Questioning: Ask open questions, clarify, restate, endorse, and invite questions. ASK-TELL-ASK
- Information organization: Preview, summarize, transition, and review the next steps.
- Empathic communication.

Box 13.8 Teaching Methods Utilized for Doctor-Patient Communication[9]

- Role-playing
- Videotaped feedback
- Experiential exercises
- Didactics

Box 13.9 Structure and Success of Communication Training Programs[1]

Communication training programs must enable clinicians to manage their own emotional distress during discussions with palliative care patients.

The training programs must provide practice for clinicians in specialized communication skills such as shared decision making and delivering bad news.

The training programs should encourage learners to assess their own performance, and obtain feedback from the trainers to improve their skills.

The sustainability of the acquired communication skills remains to be a major area in need of improvement for long-lasting efficacy of communication skills training programs.

Box 13.10 Difficult Communication Scenarios[9]

- Breaking bad news
- Discussing unanticipated (adverse) events
- Discussing prognosis and risk
- Reaching a shared (treatment) decision
- Responding to difficult emotions
- Running family meetings
- Transitioning to palliative care and end of life
- Advanced directives (allow for a natural death)

Box 13.11 Six-Step Protocol for Breaking Bad News[2,4]

1. Get the physical context right.
2. Find out how much the patient knows.
3. Find out how much the patient wants to know.
4. Share information. (Align and educate.)
5. Respond to the patient's feelings.
6. Plan and follow through.

References

1. Maguire P, Weiner JS. Communication with terminally ill patients and their families. In: Chochinov HMC, Breitbart W, eds. *Handbook of Psychiatry in Palliative Medicine*, 2nd ed. New York: Oxford University Press; 2009:157–171.
2. Baile W, Beale E. Giving bad news to cancer patients: matching process and content. *J Clin Oncol.* 2001;19:2575–2577.
3. Buckman R. *How to Break Bad News—A Guide for Healthcare Professionals.* London: Macmillan Medical; 1993.
4. Buckman R. Communication in palliative care: a practical guide. In: Doyle D, Hanks GWC, MacDonald N, eds. *Oxford Textbook of Palliative Medicine*, 2nd ed. New York: Oxford University Press; 1998:141–156.
5. Parker B, Baile W, deMoor C, et al. Breaking bad news about cancer: patients' preferences for communication. *J Clin Oncol.* 2001;19:2049–2056.
6. Smith TJ. Tell it like it is. *J Clin Oncol.* 2000;18:3441–3445.
7. Fallowfield L. Communication and palliative medicine. In: Doyle D, Hanks G, Cherny N, Calman K, eds. *Oxford Textbook of Palliative Medicine*, 3rd ed. New York: Oxford University Press; 2004:101–107.
8. Weeks JC, Cook EF, O'Day SJ, et al. Relationship between cancer patients' predictions of prognosis and their treatment preferences. *JAMA.* 1998;279:1709–1714.
9. Kissane DW, Bylund CL, Banerjee SC, et al. Communication skills training for oncology professionals. *J Clin Oncol.* 2012 Apr 10;30(11):1242–1247. doi: 10.1200/JCO.2011.39.6184. Epub 2012 Mar 12.
10. Hack TF, Degner LF, Parker PA, SCRN Communication Team. The communication goals and needs of cancer patients. *Psychooncology* 2005;14(10):831–845; discussion 846–847.

11. Casarett DJ, Quill T. "I am not ready for hospice": strategies for timely and effective hospice discussions. *Ann Intern Med.* 2007;146(6):443–449.
12. Weiner JS, Roth J. Avoiding iatrogenic harm to patient and family while discussing goals of care near the end of life. *J Palliat Med.* 2006;9(2):451–463.
13. Simpson M, Buckman R, Stewart M, et al. Doctor-patient communication: the Toronto consensus statement. *BMJ.* 1991;303:1385–1387.
14. Suchman AL, Markakis K, Beckman HB, et al. A model of empathic communication in the medical interview. *JAMA.* 1997;277:678–681.
15. SUPPORT Principal Investigators. A controlled trial to improve care for seriously ill hospitalized patients. *JAMA.* 1995:274:1591–1598.
16. Maguire P. Barriers to psychological care of the dying. *Br Med J.* 1985;291:1711–1713.
17. Maguire P. Improving communication with cancer patients. *Eur J Cancer.* 1999;35:2058–2065.
18. Fallowfield L, Lipkin M, Hall A. Teaching senior oncologists communication skills: results from phase I of a comprehensive longitudinal program in the United Kingdom. *J Clin Oncol.* 1998;16:1961–1968.
19. Weiner JS, Cole SA. Three principles to improve physician training for end of life care: overcoming emotional, cognitive, and skills barriers to communication skills with seriously ill patients. *J Palliat Med.* 2004;7(6):817–829.

Chapter 14

Grief and Bereavement

Bereavement care is an integral dimension of palliative care.[1] Knowledge of, and competence in, grief assessment is essential. Risk factors for complicated grief and routine assessment of the bereaved allow the psycho-oncologist to proactively intervene and reduce unnecessary morbidity.

Although words such as grief, mourning, and bereavement are commonly used interchangeably, the definitions in Box 14.1 may be helpful.

The expression of normal grief is evident through its emotional, cognitive, physical, and behavioral features.[4] Grief and depression lie on a biological continuum. The features listed in Box 14.2 illustrate the morbidity, both somatic and psychosocial, that is associated with bereavement.

As the patient and family journey through palliative care, the clinical phases of grief progress from anticipatory grief, through the immediate news of the death, to the stages of acute grief and, for some, the complications of bereavement (Boxes 14.3 and 14.4).

Although anticipatory grief was historically suggested to reduce postmortem grief,[10] intense distress is now well recognized as a marker of risk for complicated grief (Box 14.5).

When relatives or close friends gather to keep watch at the bedside of a dying person, they not only support the sick, but also facilitate their own subsequent adjustment. For years to come, these poignant moments will be recalled in immense detail. Thus, the sensitivity and courteous respect of health professionals is crucial (Box 14.6).[12]

The progression from acute grief to bereavement is never rigidly demarcated; rather, the two merge gradually (Box 14.7).[3,4]

The time course of mourning is proportional to the strength of attachment to the lost person and also varies with cultural expression. There is no sharply defined end point to grief. Older widows and widowers, for example, may continue to display their grief for several years,[16] which can correspond with a continuing relationship with the deceased. For some, this is a personal choice that may lead to chronic grief. The clinical task, then, is to differentiate those that remain with the spectrum of normality from those that cross the threshold of complicated grief.

Normal and abnormal responses to bereavement span a spectrum in which intensity of reaction, presence of a range of related grief behaviors, and time course determine the differentiation. Approximately 20% of bereaved individuals experience complicated or prolonged grief. There is growing evidence that prolonged grief or complicated grief is a unique condition characterized by separation distress and other symptoms, such as intense, unremitting yearning for

Box 14.1 Definitions Regarding Grief and Bereavement

- *Grief* is the emotional response associated with loss.[2] It is an inevitable dimension of our humanity, an adaptive adjustment process, and one that can be approached with courage if proper support is available.
- *Mourning* is the process of adaptation, including the cultural and social rituals prescribed as accompaniments.[3]
- *Bereavement* is the state of loss resulting from death.[4]
- *Anticipatory grief* precedes the death and results from the expectation of that event.[3]
- *Complicated grief* represents a pathological outcome involving psychological, social, or physical morbidity.[5]
- *Disenfranchised grief* represents the hidden sorrow of the marginalized, for whom there is less social permission to express many dimensions of loss.[6]

Box 14.2 Features of Normal Grief

Emotional

Periods of acute distress that may occur in waves that last for minutes at a time

Unavoidable crying

Preoccupation with thoughts about the deceased

A range of associated affects including sadness, anger, despair, anxiety, and guilt

Cognitive

Loss of concentration

Cognitive processes dominated by memories (reflected in storytelling, reminiscences, and conversations about the deceased)

Somatic

Numbness

Restlessness

Tension

Tremors

Sleep disturbance

Anorexia

Weight loss

Fatigue

Aches and pains

Behavioral

Social withdrawal

Wandering

Searching and seeking company and consolation

Physiological

Alterations of neuroendocrine functioning (e.g., dexamethasone suppression test)[7]

Immune changes (e.g., natural killer cell functioning)[8]

Impaired sleep efficiency[9]

Box 14.3 Course of Anticipatory Grief

- Generally draws the supportive family into a configuration of mutual comfort and greater closeness as they grapple with the news of the illness and its proposed management. For a time, this perturbation improves the care of the sick, until the pressures of daily life draw the family back toward their prior constellation.
- Movement back and forth between these different responsibilities is evident thereafter as news of illness progression unfolds.
- Periods of grief become interspersed with phases of contentment and happiness. When the family is engaged in home care of their dying member, their cohesion potentially increases as they share their fears, hopes, joys, and distress.
- Difficulties emerge for some families as they express their anticipatory grief.

Box 14.4 Common Difficulties That Emerge during Anticipatory Grief

Impaired coping
- Protective avoidance
- Denial of the seriousness of the threat
- Anger
- Withdrawal from involvement

*Subthreshold/mild psychiatric disorders**
- Depression
- Anxiety

* These develop gradually as individuals struggle to adapt to unwelcome changes.

Box 14.5 Role of the Psycho-oncologist in Anticipatory Grief

- Encourage the family to openly share their feelings as they go about the instrumental care of their dying family member or friend.
- Recognize the process of saying goodbye as one that evolves over time, with opportunities for reminiscence, celebration of the life and contribution of the dying person, expressions of gratitude, and completion of any unfinished business.[11]

the deceased, difficulty accepting the loss, and sense of meaninglessness, that remain elevated at 6 or more months after the loss.[17] Although complicated grief may be comorbid with other psychiatric disorders, its symptoms have been associated with negative physical and mental health outcomes, including poorer quality of life and suicidality, independent of depression.[17] The *Diagnostic and Statistical Manual of Mental Disorders*, 5th ed.[18] has listed complicated grief under

Box 14.6 Role of the Psycho-oncologist in Supporting Families during the Dying Process

- Helpfully comment on the process of dying by explaining the breathing patterns and commenting on any noises, secretions, patient reactions, and comfort.
- Normalize the experience empathically and reassure the family whenever concern develops.
- Discuss pain, reasons for medications, and skilfully predict events in order to assuage worry and build a collaborative approach to the care of the dying.
- Actively facilitate religious rituals. This includes appropriate notification of a religious minister or pastoral care worker.
- Once death has occurred, respect the body and express sympathy.
- Allow family members to spend time alone with the deceased, with regard to cultural approaches to the laying out of the body.[13]
- As concerns arise among staff members about the emotional response of the bereaved and its cultural appropriateness, consultation with an informed cultural intermediary may be helpful.
- Prescribe short-acting benzodiazepines, if desired.
- Perform a follow-up telephone call on the next day to check on coping and identify the need for continued support.
- Be aware of settings in which grief can be marginalized.[6] Do not ignore the disenfranchised in their sorrow.

the category of conditions for further study. The terms "complicated grief" and "prolonged grief" have been replaced by the term "persistent complex bereavement disorder" with proposed criteria, including most features of what has been more commonly known as complicated and prolonged grief in the palliative care literature. We have used the terms "complicated grief," "prolonged grief," and

Box 14.7 Phases in the Progression from Acute Grief to Bereavement

1. Initial numbness and sense of unreality
2. Waves of distress begin to occur as the bereaved suffer intense pining and yearning for their lost one. Memories of the deceased trigger these acute pangs of grief.
3. As the pain of separation occurs, a phase of disorganization emerges as loneliness resulting from the loss. This phase has been aptly descried as a constant background disturbance of restlessness, inattention, sadness, and despair, with social withdrawal that can last for several months.[14]
4. A phase of reorganization and recovery develops as nostalgia replaces sadness, morale improves, and an altered worldview is constructed. Personal growth can be recognized at this stage and new creativity is expressed.[15]

"persistent complex bereavement" interchangeably in this handbook because we recognize the unfamiliarity of the palliative care world around the globe with the new terminology proposed by the DSM-V (Box 14.8).

When psychiatric disorders complicate bereavement, their recognition and management is straightforward (see chapters 4–8). It is the subthreshold symptoms that present a greater clinical challenge. Studies of the bereaved indicate groups in which clusters of intense grief symptoms are distinct from

Box 14.8 Common Psychiatric Complications of Grief

- *Depression*
  - Occurs in 16% to 50% of the bereaved and gradually decreases to 15% over the 2 years following death of the loved one.[19,20]
  - The features of any major depressive episode following bereavement resemble major depression at other points of the life cycle.[21]
  - There is a tendency to chronicity, considerable social morbidity, and risk of inadequate treatment.
- *Anxiety disorders*
  - Occur in up to 30% of the bereaved[7]
  - Usually take the form of adjustment disorders, generalized anxiety disorder, and/or phobic states
  - Patients commonly present to general practitioners with a range of somatic concerns.
  - Separation anxiety of a heightened nature can be distinguished from anxiety symptoms of a general kind.
- *Alcohol abuse or other substance abuse and dependence disorders*
  - Typically an exacerbation of pre-existing psychiatric states
  - Individuals predisposed to alcohol abuse, or dependence on other substances such as benzodiazepines, tend to relapse during bereavement.[22]
  - Other family members often raise the alarm.
- *Psychotic disorders*
  - Bereavement is a common precipitant of relapse of psychotic illnesses, such as bipolar disorder or schizophrenia in predisposed individuals.
  - Mania occasionally presents for the first time in the setting of bereavement.
  - Hearing the deceased person or the illusion of having seen the deceased are common experiences of the bereaved, and should not be mistaken for psychotic disorders.
- *Post-traumatic stress disorder*
  - Palliative care deaths involving profound breakdown of bodily surfaces, gross disfigurement due to head and neck cancers, or other factors leading to loss of the patient's dignity may generate traumatic memories in the bereaved.
  - Post-traumatic stress disorder has been found to correlate with the perceived inadequacy of the "goodbye."[23] Thus, rituals to complete this farewell may be helpful when incorporated into related grief therapies.

Box 14.9 Inhibited or Delayed Grief

- Empirical studies have generally identified these avoidant forms of complicated grief in up to 5% of the bereaved.
- Although the use of avoidance may serve some as a temporary coping mechanism, its persistence is usually associated with relationship difficulties or the emergence of a hypomanic state in individuals with bipolar disorder.
- Grief may be understandably absent when there has been no bond of attachment to the deceased. Similarly, cultural variation may influence the expression of grief.
- Inhibited or delayed grief may not always present clinically, but rather, often reappears in later years as an unresolved issue.

uncomplicated grief.[24,25] Their recognition calls for an experienced clinical judgement that does not normalize the distress as understandable (Boxes 14.9–14.11).

These risk factors should be assessed at entry to the service and upgraded during the phase of palliative care, including revision shortly after the death. Caregivers with prolonged or complicated grief have been shown to underutilize mental health services; therefore, it is of utmost importance to identify those at risk for complicated or prolonged grief while the patient is still alive.[27] During the completion of the family genogram, prior losses and coping are considered. Thus, this is an ideal time to assess risk factors involving family relationships. Some palliative care services have developed checklists based on such risk factors to generate a numerical measure of risk. There has been insufficient validation of such scales at this stage, but the presence of any single factor in Box 14.12 signifies risk. Continued observation of the pattern of grief evolution over time is appropriate whenever such concern exists.

Box 14.10 Chronic Grief

- Common form of complicated grief
- Particularly associated with overly dependent relationships
- A sense of abandonment is avoided by perpetuation of the relationship through memorialization of the deceased and maintenance of continuing bonds.
- No cognitive transition is achieved in the worldview of the bereaved.
- Social withdrawal and depression are common.
- A fantasy of reunion with the deceased can cause suicide to be an increasingly attractive option.
- Appropriate treatment includes both the use of pharmacology for depression and cognitive behavioral therapy in order to reality-test the loss and promote socialization (via the scheduling of activities, etc.)

Box 14.11 Traumatic Grief

- Usually occurs when death has been unexpected or shocking in its nature (traumatic, violent, stigmatized, or perceived as undignified)
- Intensive recollections, including flashbacks, nightmares, and recurrent intrusive memories, cause hyperarousal, disbelief, insomnia, irritability, and disturbed concentration, which distorts normal grieving.[26]
- The shock of the death can precipitate mistrust, anger, detachment, and an unwillingness to accept its reality.
- These reactions, at a subthreshold level, merge with the full features of post-traumatic stress disorder. However, the subthreshold state has been observed to persist for years and to contribute to substantial morbidity.
- The DSM-V proposed criteria for the persistent complex bereavement disorder includes a "traumatic bereavement" specifier for those who lost a loved one to homicide or suicide.[18]

Because loss is ubiquitous in the palliative care setting, psycho-oncologists need skill in the application of grief therapies. The most basic model is a supportive-expressive intervention in which the person is invited to share his or her feelings about the loss to a health professional who will listen and seek to understand the other's distress in a comforting manner. The essential therapeutic aspects of this encounter are the sharing of distress and, through the relational understanding that is acknowledged, some shift in cognitive appraisal of the reality that has been forever altered (Table 14.1; Box 14.13).

Box 14.12 Risk Factors for Complicated Grief

Nature of the death

Untimely within the life cycle (e.g., death of a child)

Sudden and unexpected (e.g., death from septic neutropenia during chemotherapy)

Traumatic (e.g., shocking cachexia and disability)

Stigmatized (e.g., AIDS or suicide)

Vulnerabilities of the caregiver/bereaved

Past history of psychiatric disorder

Personality and coping style (e.g., intense worrier, low self-esteem)

Cumulative experience of losses

Nature of the relationship with the deceased

Overly dependent (e.g., clinging, symbiotic)

Ambivalent (e.g., angry and insecure with alcohol abuse, infidelity, gambling)

Family and support network

Dysfunctional family (e.g., poor cohesiveness and communication, high conflict)

Isolated (e.g., new migrant, new residential move)

Alienated (e.g., perception of poor support)

Table 14.1 Models of Grief Therapy

	Potential for Application	Indications
Supportive-expressive	Individual and/or group	Avoidance of emotional expression; inhibited or delayed grief; isolation/need of support; Established psychiatric disorder
Interpersonal or psychodynamic	Individual and/or group	Relational issues; role transition difficulties
Cognitive-behavioral	Individual and/or group	Chronic grief with intractable behaviors; traumatic grief; post-traumatic stress disorder
Family-focused	Family	At risk or clearly dysfunctional families; at-risk children or adolescents
Combined pharmacotherapy with any of the above models	Individual	Depressive disorders; anxiety disorders; sleep disorders

Pharmacotherapies are widely used to support the bereaved; nonetheless, judicious prescription is important (Table 14.2).

Family therapists have long recognized the influence of family processes on mourning and its outcomes.[31] Exploration of the association between family functioning and bereavement morbidity has highlighted the manner in which family dysfunction predicts increased rates of psychosocial morbidity in the bereaved.[32] Family-centered care that focuses on the well-being of the family during palliative care is helpful to reduce rates of morbidity in those subsequently bereaved (Box 14.14).

Box 14.13 Considerations for Interventions for Grief and Bereavement

- Intervention is not always warranted. For the majority, although bereavement is painful, their personal resilience will ensure their normal adaptation. There can therefore be no justification for routine intervention, as normal grief is not pathological.
- Those considered at risk of maladaptive outcome should be treated preventively, and those who later develop complicated bereavement need active treatments. Effective therapies are available to assist in the management of complicated grief.[28]
- Adoption of any model (or parts thereof) is predicated on the clinical issues and associated predicaments that arise. Variation will be influenced by age, perception of support, nature of the death, personal health of the bereaved, and the presence of comorbid states.
- Grief therapy tends to be focused and time limited, but multimodal therapies are commonplace.
- Group, in addition to individual therapies, better support the lonely so that socialization complements individual change.

Table 14.2 Pharmacotherapy for Complicated Grief

	Indication	Guidelines
Benzodiazepines	Anxiety Sleep disturbance	Intermittent use to avoid tachyphylaxis and dependence
Antidepressants	Depressive disorder Panic attacks Moderate to severe adjustment disorders[29,30]	Low-dose TCAs may be considered for insomnia, otherwise SSRIs or combined noradrenergic and serotonergic reuptake inhibitors are indicated
Antipsychotics	Hypomania, mania Psychosis	

Box 14.14 Family-Focused Grief Therapy[33–35]

- Aims to improve family functioning while also supporting the expression of grief
- Can be applied preventively to those families judged through screening to be at high risk of morbid outcome[34]
- Commences during palliative care and continues through the early phases of bereavement until there is confidence that morbidity has been prevented or appropriately treated
- Invites the family to identify, and agree to work on, aspects of family life that they stigmatize as problematic
- Enhances cohesion
- Promotes open communication of thoughts and feelings
- Teaches effective problem solving to reduce conflict and stigmatize tolerance of different opinions
- Improved functioning of the family as a unit becomes the means to accomplish adaptive mourning

References

1. Zisook S, Irwin S, Shear K. Understanding and managing bereavement in palliative care. In: Chochinov HMC, Breitbart W, eds. *Handbook of Psychiatry in Palliative Medicine*, 2nd ed. New York: Oxford University Press; 2009:202–219.
2. Stroebe M, Stroebe W, Hansson R, eds. *Handbook of Bereavement*. Cambridge, UK: Cambridge University Press; 1993.
3. Raphael B. *The Anatomy of Bereavement*. London: Hutchinson; 1983.
4. Parkes C. *Bereavement: Studies of Grief in Adult Life*, 3rd ed. Madison, WI: International Universities Press; 1998.
5. Rando T. *Treatment of Complicated Mourning*. Champaign, IL: Research Press; 1983.
6. Doka K. Disenfranchised grief. In Doka K, ed. *Disenfranchised Grief: Recognizing Hidden Sorrow*. Lexington, MA: Lexington Books; 1989:3–11.
7. Jacobs S, Bruce M, Kim K. Adrenal function predicts demoralisation after losses. *Psychosomatics* 1997;38:529–534.
8. Esterling B, Kiecolt-Glaser J, Glaser R. Psychosocial modulation of cytokine-induced natural killer cell activity in older adults. *Psychosomatics* 1996;38:529–534.
9. Hall M, Baum A, Buysse D, et al. Sleep as a mediator of the stress-immune relationship. *Psychosom Med*. 1998;60:48–51.
10. Parkes C. Determinants of outcome following bereavement. *Omega* 1975;6:303–323.
11. Meares R. On saying goodbye before death. *JAMA*. 1981;246:1227–1229.
12. Maguire P. Barriers to psychological care of the dying. *Br Med J*. 1985;291: 1711–1713.

13. Parkes C, Laungani P, Young B, eds. *Death and Bereavement across Cultures.* London: Routledge; 1997.
14. Hofer M. Relationships as regulators: a psychobiologic perspective on bereavement. *Psychosom Med.* 1984;46:183–197.
15. Polloch G. *The Mourning-Liberation Process.* New Haven, CT: International University Press; 1989.
16. Zisook S, Schuchter S. The first four years of widowhood. *Psychiatric Ann.* 1985;16:288–294.
17. Prigerson HG, Horowitz MJ, Jacobs SC, et al. Prolonged grief disorder: psychometric validation of criteria proposed for DSM-V and ICD-11. *PLoS Med.* 2009;6:e1000121.
18. American Psychiatric Association. *Diagnostic and Statistical Manual of Mental Disorders*, 5th ed. Arlington, VA: American Psychiatric Publishing; 2013:5–25.
19. Zisook S, Schuchter S, Sledge P. The spectrum of depressive phenomena after spousal bereavement. *J Clin Psychiatry* 1994;55:29–36.
20. Clayton P. Bereavement and depression. *J Clin Psychiatry* 1990;51:34–38.
21. Karam E. The nosological status of bereavement-related depressions. *Br J Psychiatry* 1994;165:48–52.
22. Jacobs S. *Pathological Grief.* Washington, DC: American Psychiatric Association Press, 1993.
23. Schut H, Stroebe M, de Keijser J, et al. Intervention for the bereaved: gender differences in the efficacy of two counseling programmes. *Br J Clin Psychol.* 1997;36:63–72.
24. Parkes C, Weiss R. *Recovery from Bereavement.* New York: Basic Books, 1983.
25. Prigerson H, Maciejewski P, Newson J, et al. Inventory of complicated grief. *Psychiatry Res.* 1995;59:65–79.
26. Prigerson H, Jacobs S. Traumatic Grief as a distinct disorder: A rationale, consensus criteria, and a preliminary empirical test. In Stroebe M, Hansson R, Stroebe W, Schut H, eds. *Handbook of Bereavement Research: Consequences, Coping, and Care.* Washington, DC: American Psychological Association; 2001:613–637.
27. Lichtenthal WG, Nilsson M, Kissane DW, Breitbart W, Kacel E, Jones EC, et al. Underutilization of mental health services among bereaved caregivers with prolonged grief disorder. *Psychiatric Serv.* 2011;62:10.
28. Kissane DW. Bereavement. In: Doyle D, Hanks G, Cherny N, Calman K, eds. *Oxford Textbook of Palliative Medicine*, 3rd ed. New York: Oxford University Press; 2004:1135–1154.
29. Jacobs S, Nelson J, Zisook S. Treating depressions of bereavement with antidepressants: a pilot study. *Psychiatric Clin North Am.* 1987;10:501–510.
30. Pasternak R, Reynolds C, Schlernitzauer M. Acute open-trial nortriptyline therapy of bereavement-related depression in late life. *J Clin Psychiatry.* 1991;52:307–310.
31. Kissane D, Bloch S. Family grief. *Br J Psychiatry* 1994;164:728–740.
32. Kissane D, Bloch S, Dowe D, et al. The Melbourne family grief study I & II. *Am J Psychiatry* 1996;153, 650–658, 659–666.
33. Kissane DW, McKenzie M, Bloch S, et al. Family focus grief therapy: a randomized controlled trial in palliative care and bereavement. *Am J Psychiatry* 2006;163(7):1208–1218.

34. Kissane D, Lichtenthal WG, Zaider T. Family care before and after bereavement. *J Death Dying* 2008;56(1):21–32.

35. Kissane DW, Lichtenthal WG. Family focused grief therapy: from palliative care into bereavement. *Handbook of Bereavement Research and Practice: Advances in Theory and Intervention.* Washington, DC: American Psychological Association; 2008:485–510.

Appendices

Resources for Patients and Health Care Professionals

Appendix I: Books, Websites, and Journals for Professionals and Patients

Books

Abrahm JL. *A Physician's Guide to Pain and Symptom Management in Cancer Patients.* Baltimore: John Hopkins University Press; 2000.

Altilio T, Otis-Green S, eds. *Oxford Textbook of Palliative Social Work.* New York: Oxford University Press; 2011.

American Association of Hospice and Palliative Medicine. *AAHPM Pocket Guide to Hospice/Palliative Medicine.* Glenview, IL: American Academy of Hospice and Palliative Medicine; 2003.

American Association of Hospice and Palliative Medicine. *AAHPM Unipacs 1-8: Hospice and Palliative Care Training for Physicians.* Glenview, IL: American Academy of Hospice and Palliative Medicine; 2003.

Byock I. *Dying well.* New York: Riverhead Books; 1997.

Carter BS, Levetown M, eds. *Palliative Care for Infants, Children, and Adolescents: A Practical Handbook.* Baltimore: Johns Hopkins University Press; 2004.

Chochinov HMC, Breitbart W, eds. *Handbook of Psychiatry in Palliative Medicine*, 2nd ed. New York: Oxford University Press; 2009.

Hanks GWC, Cherny N, Christakis NS, Fallon M, Kassa S, Porteoy RK, eds. *Oxford Textbook of Palliative Medicine*, 4th ed. New York: Oxford University Press; 2010.

Faull C, Richard W. *Palliative Care—an Oxford Core Text.* New York: Oxford University Press; 2002.

Ferrell B, Coyle N. *Textbook on Palliative Nursing.* New York: Oxford University Press; 2001.

Ferris F, Cummings I. *Palliative care: Towards a Consensus in Standardized Principles of Practice.* Ottawa: Canadian Palliative Care Association; 1995.

Field MJ, Cassel CK, eds. *Improving Palliative Care: We Can Take Better Care of People with Cancer.* Washington, DC: Institute of Medicine; 2003.

Foley KM, Gelband H, eds. *Institute of Medicine Report: Improving Palliative Care for Cancer.* Washington, DC: National Academy Press; 2001.

George J, Taylor GJ, Kurent JE. *A Clinician's Guide To Palliative Care.* Malden, MA: Blackwell; 2003.

Goldman A, Hain R, Liben S. *Oxford Textbook of Palliative Care for Children.* New York: Oxford University Press; 2006.

Hallenbeck J. *Palliative Care Perspectives.* New York: Oxford University Press; 2003.

Hanks G, Adam J, Addington-Hall J, Bagg J. *ABC of Palliative Care (ABC)*, 2nd ed. Glasgow: Blackwell; 2006.

Holland JC, Breitbart W, Aconsen PB, Lederberg MS, Loscalzo MJ, McCorkle R, eds. *Psycho-oncology*, 2nd ed. New York: Oxford University Press; 2010.

Lloyd-Williams M, ed. *Psychosocial Issues in Palliative Care.* New York: Oxford University Press; 2003.

Lynn J, Harrold J. *Handbook for Mortals: Guidance for People Facing Serious Illness.* New York: Oxford University Press, 1999.

MacDonald N. *Palliative Medicine: A Case Based Manual.* New York: Oxford University Press; 1998.

National Hospice Organization. Standards and Accreditation Committee: Medical Guidelines Task Force. *Medical Guidelines for Determining Prognosis in Selected Non-Cancer Diseases*, 2nd ed. Arlington, VA: National Hospice Organization; 1997.

National Research Council. *Approaching Death: Improving Care at the End of Life.* Washington, DC: Institute of Medicine; 1997.

Quill T. *Caring for Patients at End-of-Life: Facing an Uncertain Future Together.* New York: Oxford University Press; 2001.

Sims R, Moss V. *Palliative Care for People with AIDS*, 2nd ed. London: Edward Arnold, 1995.

Solomon M, Romer A, Heller K. *Innovation in End of Life Care: Practical Strategies and International Perspectives.* New York: Mary Ann Liebert; 2000.

Solomon M, Romer A, Heller K, Weissman D. *Innovation in End of Life Care: Practical Strategies and International Perspectives*, vol 2. New York: Mary Ann Liebert; 2002.

Strada A. *The Helping Professional's Guide to End-of-Life Care.* Oakland, CA: New Harbinger Publications; 2013.

Waller A, Caroline NL. *Handbook of Palliative Care in Cancer*, 2nd ed. Boston: Butterworth/Heinemann; 2000.

Watson M, Kissane D. *Handbook of Psychotherapy in Cancer Care.* West Sussex, UK: Wiley; 2011.

Woodruff R. *Palliative Medicine: Symptomatic and Supportive Care for Patients with Advanced Cancer and AIDS (3rd Ed).* Melbourne: Oxford University Press; 1999.

Websites

Americans for Better Care of the Dying	www.abcd-caring.org
Canadian Virtual Hospice Project	www.virtualhospice.ca
Center to Advance Palliative Care	www.capc.org
Certificate in Palliative Care American Board of Hospice and Palliative Medicine	www.abhpm.org
Completing a Life	completingalife.msu.edu
Data Analysis and Reports for Toolkit Instruments	www.chcr.brown.edu/dart
Dying Well	www.dyingwell.org

Education for Physicians on End-of-Life Care Curriculum	www.epec.net
End-of-Life: Exploring Death in America (NPR Series)	www.npr.org/programs/death
European School of Oncology	www.cancerworld.org
End-of-Life Physician Education Resources Center.	www.eperc.mcw.edu
Palliative Care: A self-study CME Course	
End of Life Nursing Education Consortium (ELNEC)	www.aacn.nche.edu/elnec
Hospice and Palliative Nurses Association (HPNA)	www.hpna.org
Hospice Education Institute	www.hospiceworld.org
Hospice Foundation of America	www.hospicefoundation.org
Introduction to Palliative Care Nursing Course	www.cancernursing.org
National Hospice and Palliative Care Organizations	www.nhpco.org
National Hospice Foundation	www.hospiceinfo.org
National Comprehensive Cancer Network (NCCN)	www.nccn.org/professionals/physician_gls
NCCN Clinical Practice Guidelines in Oncology-Cancer Related Fatigue, V.1.2013	www.nccn.org/professionals/physicians_gls/PDF/fatigue.pdf
Pan Canadian Practice Guideline: Screening, Assessment and Care of Cancer-Related Fatigue in Adults with Cancer	http://www.capo.ca/Fatigue_Guideline_.pdf
PBS's On Our Own Terms	www.pbs.org/wnet/onourownterms
Promoting Excellence in End-of-Life Care	www.promotingexcellence.org
Supportive Care of the Dying:	www.careofdying.org
TIME: Toolkit of Instruments to Measure EOL care	www.chcr.brown.edu/pcoc/toolkit
WHO: Palliative Care	www.who.int/cancer/palliative/en
Zen Hospice Project	www.zenhospice.org

Palliative Care Journals

European Journal of Pain
European Journal of Cancer Care
European Journal of Palliative Care
Health Policy

Home Health Care Services Quarterly
Innovations in End-of-Life Care
International Journal of Palliative Nursing
The Internet Journal of Pain, Symptom Control and Palliative Care

Journal of Cancer Pain and Symptom Palliation
Journal of Clinical Oncology
Journal of Pain and Symptom Management

Journal of HIV/AIDS and Social Services
Journal of Hospice and Palliative Nursing

Journal of Neuropathic Pain and Symptom Palliation
Journal of Pain & Palliative Care
Pharmacotherapy Journal of Palliative Care
Journal of Palliative Medicine
Journal of Psychosocial Oncology

Journal of Social Work in End of Life and Palliative Care
Journal of Social Work in Long-Term Care
Loss, Grief & Care
Medicina Paliativa (in Spanish)
Pain
Pain Advocacy Community Newsletter
Pain Reviews

Palliative and Supportive Care

Palliative Medicine
Progress in Palliative Care
Psycho-Oncology

Supportive Care in Cancer

Zeitschrift für Palliativmedizin (in German)

Appendix II: Certificate Training Programs

Center for Palliative Care Education
(depts.washington.edu/pallcare)
Northwest AIDS Education and Training Center
University of Washington
Seattle, WA

Certificate in Palliative Care

www.palliumwales.co.uk
University of Wales
College of Medicine Palliative Care Education Unit
United Kingdom
Ph: 44 (0) 29 2019 6112/11

Diploma in Palliative Care
Coventry University
United Kingdom
Marketing and Admissions Unit: Ph: 44 (0) 24 7679 5959
E-mail: hssgen@coventry.ac.uk

Diploma in Palliative Care Course
University of Gloucestershire
School of Health & Social Sciences
Francis Close Hall, Swindon Road
Cheltenham, Gloucestershire GL50 4AZ
United Kingdom
Ph: 44 01242 536197; Fax: 44 01242 543234
E-mail: shss@glos.ac.uk

Diploma in Supportive and Palliative Care
Sheffield Hallam University
City Campus, Howard Street,
Sheffield S1 1WB
United Kingdom
Ph: 44 0114 225 5555

Master of Science in Palliative Care
Flinders University
GPO Box 2100
Adelaide SA 5001
Australia
General Information: International students should contact:
Ph: (+ 618) 8201 2727; Fax: (+ 618) 8201 3177

Master of Science in Palliative Care
King's College London
Department of Palliative Care and Policy
United Kingdom
Ph: 44 (0) 20 7848 5584
E-mail: jonathan.s.koffman@kcl.ac.uk

Palliative Care in HIV Management
Global AIDS Learning & Evaluation Network (GALEN)
International Association of Physicians in AIDS Care (IAPAC)
http://www.hospicecare.com/resources/pdf-docs/galen-pallcare-eng.pdf

Palliative Care Research: Strategic Training Program
A joint initiative by Universite Laval, McGill University, University of Ottawa,
Canadian Institutes of Health Research,
National Cancer Institute of Canada
Canada
Ph: (514) 735-1347; Fax (514) 735-1074
E-mail: saode.savary@mcgill.ca

Appendix III: Palliative Care Organizations

International Organizations

International Association for Hospice and Palliative Care (IAHPC)
www.hospicecare.com
5535 Memorial Drive, Suite F
PMB 509
Houston, TX 77007

International Association for the Study of Pain (IASP)
www.iasp-pain.org
900 NE 43rd Street, Suite 306
Seattle, WA 98105-6020

International Observatory on End-of-Life Care (IOELC)
www.eolc-observatory.net
Lancaster University, Institute for Health Research
Bowland Tower East, Alexandra Square
Lancaster, LA1 4YT
United Kingdom

International Union Against Cancer (UICC)
www.uicc.org
62 route de Frontenex
1207 Geneva
Switzerland

Africa

African Palliative Care Association (APCA)
www.apca.co.ug
Hospice Africa Uganda
PO Box 7757
Kampala
Uganda

Foundation for Hospices in Sub-Saharan Africa (FHSSA)
www.fhssa.org
1700 Diagonal Road, Suite 630
Alexandria, VA 22314

Hospice Palliative Care Association of South Africa
www.hospicepalliativecaresa.co.za
PO Box 28391
Danhof 9310 Free State Africa

Americas

American Academy of Hospice and Palliative Medicine (AAHPM)
www.aahpm.org
PO Box 14288
Gainesville, FL 32604-2288

American Board of Hospice and Palliative Medicine (ABHPM)
www.abhpm.org
9200 Daleview Court
Silver Spring, MD 20901

Association for Death Education and Counseling (ADEC)
www.adec.org
342 North Main Street
West Hartford, CT 06117-2507

Association Latinoamericana de Cuidados Palliativos (ALCP)
www.cuidadospaliativos.org
c/o Dr. Roberto Wenk
Juncal 860
Buenos Aires, 1062
Argentina

Canadian Hospice Palliative Care Association (CHPCA)
www.chpca.net
Saint-Vincent Hospital, Annex B
60 Cambridge Street North
Ottawa, ON K1R 7A5
Canada

Caring Connections—program of NHPCO
www.caringinfo.org

Children's Hospice International
www.chionline.org
901 North Pitt Street, Suite 230
Alexandria, VA 22314

National Hospice and Palliative Care Organization (NHPCO)
www.nhpco.org
1700 Diagonal Road, Suite 625
Alexandria, VA 22314

Pan American Health Organization/Regional WHO Office
www.paho.org
525 23rd Street, North West
Washington, DC 20037

Asia-Pacific

Asia-Pacific Hospice Palliative Care Network (APHN)
www.aphn.org
Department of Palliative Medicine/National Cancer Center
11 Hospital Drive
Singapore 169610
Singapore

AustralAsian Palliative Care Link International (APLI)
www.petermac.org
Peter MacCallum Cancer Institute, Pain and Palliative Care Services
Locked Bag 1/ A Backett Street
Victoria, 8006
Australia

Australian & New Zealand Society of Palliative Medicine, Inc.
www.anzspm.org.au
PO Box 2918
Cheltenham
Victoria, 3192
Australia

Beijing Living Will Promotion Association
http://www.xzyzy.com/index.html

"Heart of Gold" National Hospice Service Program
http://www.hospice.com.cn/

Li Ka Shing Foundation
Shantou University Medical College
22 Xinling Road
Shantou, Guangdong, 515041
China

Hospice New Zealand
www.hospice.org.nz
PO Box 12481
Wellington
New Zealand

Malaysian Hospice Council
www.sabah.org/my/mhc
c/o Rumah Hospis
250A Jalan Air Itam
10460 Penang
Malaysia

National Council for Hospice / Palliative Care
Philippine Cancer Society
310 San Rafael St.
San Miguel, 1005
Manila
Philippines

Pain and Palliative Care Society
www.painandpalliativecare.org/homepagefiles/ipmintro
Medical College (PO)
Calicut 673008,
Kerala
India

Palliative Care Australia
www.pallcare.org.au
PO Box 55
Yarralumla ACT 2600
Australia

Peace House Hospice
1000-1, Inokuchi,
Nakai, Ashigarakami
Kanagawa 259-0151
Japan

Society for the Promotion of Hospice Care
www.hospicecare.org.hk
The Committee of Rehabilitation and Palliative Care, China (CRPC)
No. 1095 Liberation Road,
Qiaokou District, Wuhan,
Hubei Province, 430030
China

Europe

Eastern and Central Europe Palliative Task Force (ECEPT)
www.oncology.am.poznan.pl/ecept/emenu.php
Karol Marcinkowski University
Ul Lakowa ½
Poznan, 61878
Poland

European Association for Palliative Care (EAPC)
www.eapcnet.org
National Cancer Institute
Via Venezian 1
Milan 20133
Italy

European Organization for Research and Treatment of Cancer (EORTC)
www.eortc.be

Help the Hospices
www.helpthehospices.org.uk
Hospice House
34-44 Britannia Street
London, WC1X 9JG
United Kingdom

Palliative Care in Central and Eastern Europe and
Former Soviet Union Countries
www.hospice.hu

UK Forum for Hospice and Palliative Care
www.helpthehospices.org.uk
Hospice House
34-44 Britannia Street
London, WC1X 9JG
United Kingdom

Psycho-Oncology Societies*

International Psycho-Oncological Society
www.ipos-society.org
c/o Custom Management Group
2365 Hunters Way
Charlottesville, VA 22911
Ph: 1 434.293.5350; Fax: 1 434.977.1856

* There are close to 60 national psycho-oncology societies worldwide, many of which can be accessed through the IPOS website: www.ipos-society.org.

Index

Tables and boxes are indicated by an italic *t* or *b* following the page number, respectively.

Q